The
BRAIN
DISORDERS
SOURCEBOOK

D0113155

Also by Roger S. Cicala, M.D.:

The Heart Disease Sourcebook

The

BRAIN
DISORDERS
SOURCEBOOK

Roger S. Cicala, M.D.

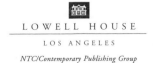

LOWELL HOUSE

LOS ANGELES

NTC/Contemporary Publishing Group

Library of Congress Cataloging-in-Publication Data

Cicala, Roger.
    The brain disorders sourcebook / Roger S. Cicala.
        p.   cm.
    Includes index.
    ISBN 0-7373-0093-0
    1. Brain—Diseases Popular works. 2. Cerebrovascular disease
Popular works. 3. Brain—Tumors Popular works. I. Title
RC386.2.C53 1999
616.8—dc21   99-15345
                                                         CIP

Published by Lowell House.
A division of NTC/Contemporary Publishing Group, Inc.
4255 West Touhy Avenue, Lincolnwood, Illinois 60646-1975 U.S.A.

Design by Kate Mueller, Electric Dragon Productions.
Illustrations by Roger S. Cicala.

Printed in the United States of America
International Standard Book Number: 0-7373-0093-0
    00 01 02 03 04 DHD 18 17 16 15 14 13 12 11 10 9 8 7 6 5 4 3 2

CONTENTS

INTRODUCTION

In many ways, diseases that affect our brains are more frightening than diseases affecting other parts of our bodies. Any major illness can limit our activities, cause us pain or suffering, and even cause death. Diseases affecting our brain, however, truly affect "us." They may change the way we think, remember, or handle our emotions. They can even alter our personality. If I break my arm, my ability to perform certain tasks and care for myself is going to be compromised for a while. A neurological (affecting the nervous system) disease, however, may affect everything about me.

Most people have a good understanding of diseases that affect the body's major organs. We understand heart attacks, for example, and know roughly what the possible outcomes are when a loved one suffers from such a disease. Everyone has a rough idea of what a "treadmill test" and a coronary bypass operation entail. Few people outside the medical profession have a good understanding of neurologic disease, however. Most people know that a stroke can cause paralysis, but few have a good understanding of how much improvement may occur after a stroke, or what other affects it can have on the body.

When you or someone you love is affected by a neurological disease, it's almost impossible to get enough time alone with your doctor to have all of your questions answered. Even if you do, you may forget to ask an important question until after you have left the office.

This book should not only answer most of the questions you have, but it should provide you with the basic facts needed to be able to ask your doctor(s) specific questions, and more importantly to understand their answers.

If someone you love is affected by one of the specific diseases discussed in this book, you will probably want to read the chapters about that problem right away. That's fine. You'll certainly get some useful information quickly that way. Thoroughly understanding any disease affecting the brain can be an almost overwhelming task, however, unless we understand the way the normal brain functions. For this reason *I strongly urge you to go back and read the first section of the book that discusses the structure and function of the normal brain.* This section also explains all the different tests that are used to diagnose a neurological disease.

Once you understand the structure and function of the normal brain, it becomes much easier to understand why a disease causes certain symptoms and not others. If you now return to the specific chapters concerning the disease affecting yourself or your loved one, you will find it easier to understand how the disease may progress, or how much recovery might take place. The specific chapters will also provide a complete list of the treatments that might be effective for a given disease, as well as the risks and side effects associated with each treatment.

Any medical information book, including this one, will have its limitations. It can't answer all your questions, or offer comfort as your loved one struggles with a serious disease. There are many organizations that can do just that, however, and the appendices list support groups and research institutes for almost every type of neurological disease. I urge you to contact an appropriate support group. They can provide even more information and ease any fears you might have about the disease in question.

ACKNOWLEDGMENTS

My nearly grown children Kristin and Drew (el Guapo) continue to tolerate endless hours of Dad "typing his books." Actually, now that they're teenagers, they seem almost suspiciously supportive of me spending hours in the office. As long as I don't tie up a phone line.

Thanks to my parents, without whose continued support, help, and a few choice words I would probably have followed my first career choice (rock star) instead of medicine. Special thanks to my coworkers: Cindy, Dana, Christie, Ami, Tammy, Ginger, and Kathy who put up with my irritability whenever I'm behind on deadlines. And to my editors, Bud and Maria, who exhibited (nearly) endless patience during those same times.

PART I

The Structure and Function of the Brain

CHAPTER 1

The Anatomy
of the Brain

The human brain is incredibly complex in both its structure and function. Most of you will probably skip this chapter when you first pick up this book and go straight to the section that describes the neurologic problem you are most interested in. That's fine, but you should eventually wander back here. It's almost impossible to understand why the brain isn't working properly, or what symptoms a disease will cause, without having a good understanding of how the brain is organized and what it actually does.

This chapter will describe the parts that comprise the brain in some detail. It will also discuss in lesser detail the major functions of each part of the brain. More detailed descriptions of how the brain actually works are found in chapter 3, but unless you already know the basics of the brain's anatomy, it is very difficult to understand how it works. This isn't an easy subject to grasp, but it is extremely important if you truly want to understand any of the diseases that affect the brain.

And although I'll do my very best to keep this discussion organized and logical, it's easy to get lost when covering a subject this complex. Most people will find they have to go back and reread parts

of this chapter as the discussion unfolds. As my neuroanatomy pro-
fessor told me in medical school, "You can't understand any part of
the brain's structure and function until you understand all of the
brain's structure and function." It's sort of a medical catch-22, but one
that makes sense when you consider that although each part of the
brain has a primary purpose, it is also totally interconnected and de-
pendent upon other parts of the brain.

The Brain's Cells

THE NEURONS

The major brain cell from the point of view of function (although not
the most numerous type of cell in the brain) is the neuron, or nerve
cell. Neurons come in a variety of shapes and sizes, but each has the
same basic structure (Fig. 1.1) and function. Each neuron is comprised of a thick cell body (the part of the cell containing the basic cellular structures), one or more thin filaments called dendrites, and a
single branching filament called the axon.

Function of the Neuron

The special function of all neurons is this: They are capable of transmitting an electrical-chemical message to other cells. Describing this
message in its simplest form, the neuron receives a chemical signal at
the dendrite that starts an electrical current within the neuron. The
charge passes along the entire length to the end of the axon. The neuron functions much like a wire on a circuit board, carrying current
from one place to another.

The chemical part of the message occurs at the end of the axon.
Each axon ends very close to another cell (in the brain the other cell
is another neuron). There is a small, tightly bound gap, called a
synapse, between the end of the axon and the next cell. When the

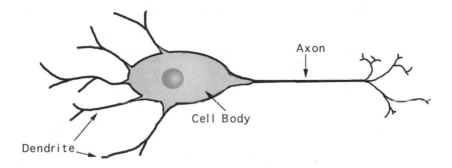

Figure 1.1   Structure of a typical neuron.

electrical message reaches the end of the axon, it releases specific chemicals, called neurotransmitters, into the synapse. Receptors on the next cell sense these chemicals, and if the receptors are stimulated strongly enough, the next cell will start its own electrical impulse.

This simple type of transmission becomes the incredibly complex process that results in a functioning brain for three main reasons. The first reason is that the chemical transmission across the synapse is not an all or nothing signal. That is, stimulation of one synaptic junction will not make the next cell start an electrical impulse. A single neuron may receive signals at hundreds or even thousands of different locations along its dendrites and on its cell body. Only when the total stimulation from all of them reaches a certain threshold will the cell create an electrical impulse.

The second reason is that a chemical transmitter can be "exciting" or "inhibiting." Some chemical messages tell a certain cell to send an electrical impulse while others tell it not to. If a cell receives both a lot of exciting signals and a lot of inhibiting signals, it probably will not send a message. If it receives only a few exciting signals, but no inhibiting signals, it probably will send a message.

The third reason is that connections between nerve cells are incredibly complex and varied. As mentioned, a single nerve cell may receive messages at thousands of different locations along its dendrites. Similarly, its axon may branch so that it sends messages to dozens of other cells. In fact, a single neuron may have 10,000 side branches.

Then consider the fact that there are about 100 million neurons in every square inch of brain surface, or approximately 100 billion neurons in the entire brain. It has been estimated that there are 500 trillion (500,000,000,000) total connections made between the neurons in the brain. And each of the 500 trillion connections can send a signal between 100 and 1,000 times a second!

For comparison, the really powerful computer I'm using to write this book can send only 300,000 instructions each second, and at best perform a meager 32 instructions at once.

Organization of Neurons in the Brain

The parts of the neuron necessary to keep it alive and functioning are located in the cell body. Although neurons don't normally divide and reproduce in human adults, they are capable of growing and repairing themselves as long as the cell body remains alive. This is part of the reason why some people who have nerve or brain damage can improve with time, while others do not. If the cell body of the neuron survives it can grow new axons and dendrites, thus reestablishing its old connections. If the cell body is killed there is no chance of a new neuron forming.

The cell bodies of many neurons are located near each other in groups, while large bundles of axons and dendrites travel together from one part of the brain to another. Since the cell bodies have a gray color, the large groups of neurons are called the "gray matter" of the brain. The axons and dendrites tend to be covered by fatty sheaths, similar to the insulation of a wire. Because fat has a white appearance, areas of the brain that consist of bundles of axons and dendrites appear white and are called the "white matter."

The brain's outside layer consists almost entirely of gray matter and is called the cortex. Overall, this layer is about 100 neurons thick. Examined under a microscope, the cortex is usually organized so that the neurons form about six distinct layers. In general, the neurons in the innermost layers send and receive signals to and from other parts of the brain, while the outer layers process incoming signals and decide what outgoing signals will be sent.

The brain's interior consists of different bundles of white matter, known as tracts, and some large areas of gray matter, known as nuclei. When a tract leaves the brain (or spinal cord for that matter) to go to structures outside the nervous system, it becomes a nerve. The larger tracts, however, are those that connect the different areas within the brain. The largest of these, known as the corpus callosum, connects the two halves of the brain.

THE GLIAL CELLS

There are an incredible number of neurons in the brain, but most of the cells within the brain are not neurons. For every neuron, there are three or more glial cells that support the neurons and give structure to the brain itself. These cells are not of major importance to our understanding of the brain, but *are* important concerning disease. It is glial cells, rather than neurons, that give rise to most forms of brain cancer.

The three main types of glial cells are oligodendrocytes (even most doctors can't pronounce it), astrocytes, and microglia. Oligodendrocytes form the fatty sheaths that cover axons and dendrites in the tracts and nerves. Astrocytes form the latticework structure that supports neurons within the brain and also help regulate the chemical balance of the brain. They also are responsible for forming scars when a part of the brain has been damaged. Microglia are the infection-fighting cells of the brain.

The Major Structures of the Brain

The microscopic neurons of the brain are organized according to a general pattern that is the same in every person. In general, neurons in the same area work together to perform roughly the same type of function or to control a single part of the body.

THE BRAIN STEM AND SPINAL CORD

The spinal cord is like the thick trunk of phone wires coming into a large building. Much of the information that enters the brain comes through the spinal cord from millions of sensory nerves located throughout the body. These nerves carry not only consciously sensed information, such as the presence of a hot burner near your fingertip, but millions of bits of information you can't consciously sense, such as how tightly your blood vessels are constricted.

Not surprisingly, given its function, the spinal cord consists largely of white matter tracts—long axons (some as long as four feet) that carry information between the distant parts of the body and the brain. The cell bodies of these neurons are located either in the center of the spinal cord in an H-shaped area of gray matter, or in small nuclei in nerves outside the spinal cord. Nerves leave the spinal cord between each of the vertebrae (backbones) to carry signals to the body.

At the point where the spinal cord enters the skull it widens to become the medulla, or brain stem (Figs. 1.2 and 1.3). The medulla is thicker than the spinal cord, and rather than being round has several bulges along its length. Additionally, several very thick nerves leave its surface. Since these nerves pass directly out through openings of the

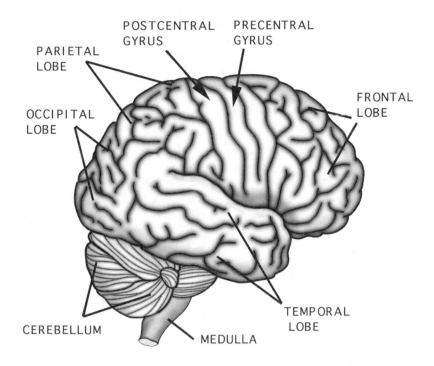

Figure 1.2 Lateral view of the brain and brain stem.

skull, rather than through the spinal cord, they (and other nerves leaving the brain directly) are called the cranial nerves (Table 1.1; Fig. 1.3). In general, the cranial nerves leaving the medulla go to the muscles of the neck, the tongue, and the inside of the mouth and throat. Another very large cranial nerve, called the vagus nerve, leaves the medulla and goes to all the internal organs in the chest, abdomen, and pelvis.

The inside of the medulla is an incredibly confusing and complex array of nuclei (areas of gray matter) and tracts (areas of white matter). This is not surprising since the axons from the spinal cord must pass through the medulla on their way to and from the brain, while at the same time the cranial nerves leaving the medulla each have nuclei

Table 1.1   The Cranial Nerves:
             Nerves That Connect Directly to the Brain

Nerve Number	Name	Function	Enters Brain At
I	Olfactory	Smell	Cerebrum
II	Optic	Vision	Cerebrum
III	Oculomotor	Eye movements	Pons
IV	Trochlear	Eye movements	Pons
V	Trigeminal	Face Sensation	Pons
VI	Abducens	Eye movements	Pons/Medulla
VII	Facial	Facial Muscles	Pons/Medulla
VIII	Acoustic	Hearing; sense of balance	Pons/Medulla
IX	Glossopharyngeal	Taste sensation; swallowing	Medulla
X	Vagus	Control of internal organs	Medulla
XI	Accessory	Neck and shoulder muscles	Medulla
XII	Hypoglossal	Tongue movement	Medulla

for their cell bodies. Additionally, the medulla controls many of the "unconscious" functions of the body, such as regulating blood pressure and breathing. Because so many different structures pass through the medulla, even a tiny area of damage in this part of the brain can cause severe symptoms.

THE PONS

Appearing to sit on top of the medulla is a large, almost round structure known as the pons (Fig. 1.3). On its surface, the pons has obvious lateral fibers that wrap around to connect it to the cerebellum through very thick tracts. The pons also has several cranial nerves

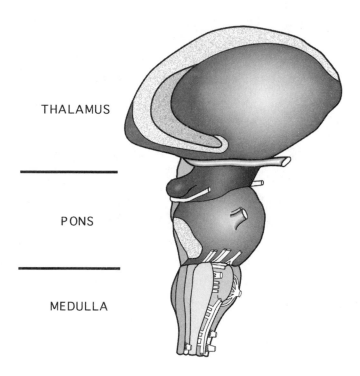

THALAMUS

PONS

MEDULLA

Figure 1.3 Lateral view of the brain stem with the cerebral hemispheres and cerebellum removed.

leaving its surface including those that provide all the sensation and motor functions of the face.

Like the medulla, the interior of the pons is crowded with tracts passing back and forth between the brain and spinal cord, as well as nuclei of its cranial nerves. Additionally, the pons has several very large nuclei and tracts that carry and process messages to and from the cerebellum. As is the case with the medulla, a small amount of damage to the pons can cause widespread problems. Damage here is more likely to affect motor functions resulting in paralysis or tremors, and less likely to cause problems with internal organs than would damage in the medulla.

THE CEREBELLUM

The cerebellum sits on the back of the pons and underneath the major parts of the brain, looking almost like a late attachment (Figs. 1.2 and 1.4). The surface of the cerebellum is covered by multiple grooves and ridges. When cut open, the interior of the cerebellum is seen to consist of a thick cortex surrounding central tracts that pass back and forth to the pons.

The function of the cerebellum is apparent if you trace its tracts. In general, all motor impulses between the brain and muscles in the body pass through the cerebellum for further processing. It is here that the brain's ideas to execute an action are fine tuned. For example, when you decide to turn a page in this book the part of your brain controlling your hand sends a message for it to move, grasp the page, and turn it. The cerebellum automatically adjusts the messages to the muscle fibers so that your hand stops smoothly at the page, rather than wavering back and forth. It also helps to regulate how much force you use so that you don't tear the page out of the book. Similarly, the cerebellum unconsciously regulates the muscles around your eye so that they automatically follow the words across the page. You don't have to think "move right one word" every tenth of a second; the cerebellum takes care of that automatically.

Damage to the cerebellum can cause a variety of problems with movement; the exact problem depends on the area affected. Diseases that cause a tremor, interfere with coordinated walking, or interfere with the coordination of fine movements of the hand are often caused by damage to, or abnormal function of, the cerebellum.

THE MIDBRAIN (THALAMUS) AND PITUITARY

The midbrain sits atop the pons, but is difficult to see because it is buried deep between the cerebral hemispheres (Fig. 1.5). The major portion of the midbrain, called the thalamus, consists of areas of gray

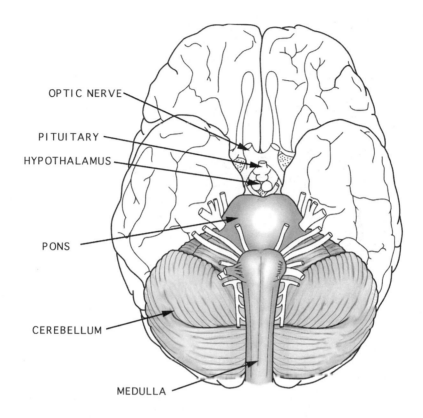

Figure 1.4   Inferior (from below) view of the brain.

matter separated and surrounded by tracts going to and from the cerebral hemispheres. The thalamus has many important functions, especially concerning automatic regulation of the body. Together with the brain stem, the thalamus regulates consciousness and sleep. It also controls sex drive and, to some extent, emotion.

Just in front of and below the thalamus is the hypothalamus. This area works with the thalamus to regulate body temperature and hunger. It also controls much of the body's functions. The hypothalamus has a small projection called the pituitary gland. This gland

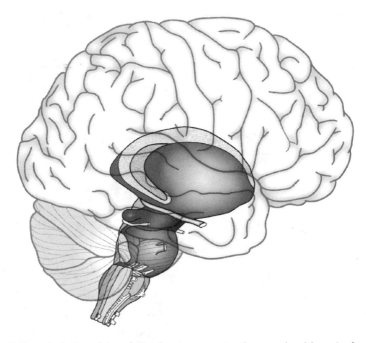

Figure 1.5   Relationship of the brain stem to the cerebral hemispheres.

secretes almost a dozen different hormones that regulate the function of most of the other glands in the body. Hypothalamic hormones regulate the monthly hormonal cycle of women, control the amount of cortisone the body manufactures, regulate blood pressure, and perform many other functions.

Just below the hypothalamus the large nerves from the eyeballs cross over each other on their way to the back of the brain (Fig. 1.4). Tumors of the pituitary gland can press on these nerves, and changes in vision are often the first symptoms of pituitary tumors. In this same area, nerves from the nose pass into areas of the brain near the thalamus that process the sense of smell. Some people believe that this connection allows the sense of smell to directly affect mood and emotion and claim they can use certain odors to treat depression and other emotional problems (aromatherapy).

THE CEREBRUM

The part of the brain most people consider to be the "real" brain is the cerebrum, which consists of the two cerebral hemispheres (Fig. 1.2). The surface of the cerebral cortex is comprised of gray matter, while the interior consists mostly of white matter (fibers that connect one area of the brain to anothers). The cerebral hemispheres are much larger than the rest of the brain combined. It is the cerebrum that differentiates humans from animals. Even simple creatures have a brain stem, cerebellum, and midbrain. Many also have a cerebrum of some kind, but only humans and a few other intelligent animals have a large cerebrum.

The two cerebral hemispheres are not entirely separate. They are connected to each other by a thick band of nerve tracts called the corpus callosum and several other tracts, each carrying messages from one side of the brain to the other. The cerebral hemispheres wrap around the midbrain, and many other tracts connect the two hemispheres to the midbrain and lower parts of the brain.

The most notable features of the cerebrum's surface are the thick twisted structures bulging from the surface, giving the appearance of hills and valleys (Fig. 1.2). The hills are called gyri and the valleys sulci. Although each individual may have a slightly different appearance to their gyri and sulci, overall they are similar enough in everyone so that they can be labelled accurately.

This labelling is important because different areas of the cortex have specific functions. Again, while there is a bit of variation in each individual, the general function of each area of the brain is known and is the same in everyone. For example, the precentral gyrus (gyrus is the singular form of gyri) controls the motor (movement) functions of the body, while the postcentral gyrus receives sensations (Fig. 1.2).

Using the most obvious landmarks, the surface of each cerebral hemisphere can effectively be divided into lobes, which are simply broad regions of the brain. The major lobes of the cerebrum are the

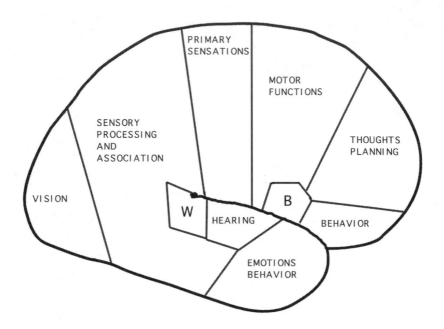

Figure 1.6   The functions of various areas of the cerebral hemispheres.
Note: Only the dominant (usually the left) hemisphere contains Broca's area (B) and Wernicke's area (W).

frontal, temporal, parietal, and occipital lobes (Fig. 1.2). The precentral gyrus and the area near it in the frontal lobe control motor function throughout the body. The remainder of the frontal lobe plays an important part in our memory, intelligence, concentration, temper, and personality (Fig. 1.6). The postcentral gyrus and areas just behind and below it receive and process sensations from various parts of the body. Certain areas in the parietal lobe and part of the temporal lobe process hearing and speech. The front of the temporal lobe is involved in memory and has some influence on emotions. The back of the occipital lobe receives input from the eyes and is responsible for "seeing."

Within each area, the brain is further organized and subdivided. If we move along the precentral gyrus from top to bottom, for example, we find areas of the brain that control, in order, the feet, legs, trunk, arms, hands, and face. Not surprisingly, only a small area of the prefrontal gyrus controls the entire trunk while very large areas control the hands and face.

The fibers that leave the cerebrum to go to the body cross from one side to the other as they pass through the brain stem. The cranial nerves that leave the brain directly do not cross over, however. Because of this, the left side of your brain controls the left side of your face and the right side of your body, and vice versa.

There are some specific differences between the left and right cerebral hemispheres. The left hemisphere is usually considered the dominant hemisphere because it controls the right hand and most people are right-handed. Neurologically, however, the dominant hemisphere is the one containing the two centers that control speech and language. In the vast majority of people, these centers are located in the left brain. In about one-third of left-handed people (about 3 percent overall), the speech centers are located on the right side of the brain.

Each hemisphere has areas that control the muscles on one side of the tongue, jaw, and throat. The dominant hemisphere also contains Broca's area, which directs those muscles to form the sounds that make up words. It also contains Wernicke's area, located in the temporal lobe, which processes sounds that are heard as understandable words (Fig. 1.6). If Broca's area becomes damaged, the affected person can make any type of sound but can't put them together to form words. If Wernicke's area is damaged, the sounds of speech are heard, but the affected person cannot understand the spoken words.

The nondominant hemisphere (usually the right) is more active in processing images and spatial facts, such as distance, angles, and perception. It's the right brain that decides if you can fit into that parking space, or if a ledge is too high to jump down from safely. It also contains areas that process musical sounds and is probably more active in emotional activities than the dominant hemisphere is.

CHAPTER 2

How the Body Protects and Supports the Brain

The brain is the most important organ of the body. People can have significant damage to their heart, liver, kidneys, or other organs and still live fairly normal lives. Even minor damage to the brain, however, significantly interferes with a person's ability to function and perform even the simplest everyday tasks. Six weeks after a heart attack (destruction of some of the heart's tissue), most people are back at work, appearing as healthy as ever. Six weeks after a stroke (destruction of some of the brain's tissue), most people are in daily therapy trying to relearn everyday functions.

Not surprisingly, the brain is more completely protected than any other organ in the body. Not only is it totally encased within the bones of the skull, it is also surrounded and supported by layers of tough connective tissue and floats in a bath of liquid to cushion it from any possible bumps and bruises that might occur.

Since brain cells are always working (even when we're asleep), the brain requires an enormous amount of blood to supply oxygen and nutrients. The brain receives more blood flow than any other organ and is supplied by a whole series of large arteries interconnected by a network of smaller blood vessels. Even the blood vessels themselves are constructed differently than those in other parts of the body, protecting the brain against toxins and other potentially damaging substances.

The structures that protect and support the brain can also cause problems at times, however. The skull is made from relatively thin bones that can turn into sharp fragments if they are fractured. The coverings of the brain can give rise to tumors as can the blood vessels. If the liquid bath surrounding the brain doesn't drain properly, it can apply enough pressure to the brain to damage the neurons. And if the blood vessels become obstructed, a stroke results.

The Skull and Meninges

The skull is not a single bone; it consists of a number of bones fitted together like a puzzle. The cranium, or part of the head above eyebrow level, is composed of several thin, sheetlike bones. In a newborn these bones are separated, but they fuse together during childhood. Because most brain growth occurs in early childhood (a one-year-old's skull is 75 percent as large as an adult's), the bones are completely fused by age eight or nine.

A skull fracture usually involves the bones of the cranium both because these bones are relatively thin and because this area is the most likely to suffer from an impact. A depressed skull fracture means that a piece of bone has been driven down toward the brain. This may simply cause a bruise on the brain's surface, or it may tear brain tissue resulting in permanent brain damage.

The base of the skull is comprised of the bones of the face and several other bones that form the bottom of the skull. These bones are quite a bit thicker than those of the cranium. Unlike the cranium, however, there are many openings through the bones of the skull base that allow both the brain's blood vessels and the cranial nerves to enter and leave the interior of the skull. These openings are called foramen. Each has its own name, or may be referred to by the structure that passes through it.

Fractures to bones in the base of the skull (basilar skull fracture) are much less common than fractures of the cranium. When they do occur, however, they can be quite dangerous because they may involve one or more of the foramen, tearing the structures that pass through the openings. Basilar skull fractures can also allow infection to enter the brain from the sinuses or may allow the fluid surrounding the brain to leak out.

The meninges are layers of connective tissue that line the inside of the skull and cover and protect the brain. Three different layers comprise it. The outermost layer is a tough sheet of leathery tissue called the dura mater. The middle layer of the meninges is made up of delicate, elastic tissue and blood vessels of different sizes and is referred to as the arachnoid layer. "Arachnoid" is a Latin word meaning spider, and this layer was so named because when examined during autopsy it has the appearance of a web rather than a single sheet of tissue. In life, however, it is really more of a fluid-filled space than an actual layer of tissue. The innermost layer of the meninges, the pia mater, tightly covers the brain's entire surface. Pia mater has many blood vessels that run along its surface, sending branches deep into the brain tissue.

The meninges themselves rarely cause any problems although they can give rise to certain types of tumors known as meningiomas. Occasionally, particularly in childhood, an infection of the meninges occurs, commonly called meningitis or spinal meningitis.

Cerebrospinal Fluid

The brain floats in a bath of salt water known as cerebrospinal fluid. The cerebrospinal fluid serves as a cushion for the brain, allowing it to float within the skull avoiding the shocks and jars from most minor bumps and injuries. It also provides some nutrients and special chemicals to the cells of the brain and serves as a conduit for the transfer of chemicals from the blood to the brain cells.

The fluid is produced in several large hollow spaces within the brain called ventricles. It flows through the ventricles and into the space between the arachnoid and pia layers of the meninges, the subarachnoid space. The fluid fills the subarachnoid space flowing around the brain and down along the spinal cord. The fluid circulates constantly and is reabsorbed by specialized areas in the arachnoid space.

An adult only has about 150 ml (less than a cup) of cerebrospinal fluid in their body at any one time, but produces and reabsorbs three times this amount each day. A condition known as hydrocephalus, or "water on the brain," results when there is too much cerebrospinal fluid. Hydrocephalus can occur if the production of fluid is too high, or if the reabsorbing mechanism doesn't work well. In most cases, however, hydrocephalus is caused by a blockage of normal fluid flow in the subarachnoid space, which prevents reabsorption from occurring. The blockage may be caused by a tumor, birth defect, or any of several less common causes.

Whatever the cause of blockage, because fluid is produced continually and the skull cannot expand (at least in adults), pressure builds up and compresses the brain. The symptoms of increased spinal fluid pressure can include headaches, vomiting, drowsiness, and confusion. Sometimes the blockage can be removed, but if not, a shunt (a surgically implanted tube) can be placed to drain the extra fluid away from the brain.

The Blood Vessels of the Brain

Learning about the anatomy of the brain's blood supply intimidates many medical students, and certainly a detailed study of the dozens of arteries supplying the brain is not appropriate for this book. Nevertheless, anyone who wants to understand how a stroke affects the brain has to know at least a little bit about the brain's blood supply. A stroke results whenever the blood supply to one part of the brain is stopped, resulting in the death of all the brain cells in that area. Since each of the brain's arteries supplies a certain area of the brain, knowing their anatomy allows us to predict what will occur when a particular artery is blocked.

The majority of blood flowing to the brain passes through the two large carotid arteries found on either side of the neck. The carotids are among the largest arteries in the body; each is as large as your little finger. Although the carotid arteries are located deep in the neck, you can feel their pulse just under the angle of your jaw. At this location the carotid splits in two. One branch, the external carotid artery, carries blood to the face and mouth. The other branch, the internal carotid artery, passes through an opening in the skull to supply blood to the brain.

The remainder of the brain's blood supply arrives via two smaller arteries, called the vertebral arteries. These pass into the bones of the neck and flow up the spine to enter the skull along with the spinal cord. They follow along either side of the medulla and come together on the front of the pons to form the single basilar artery. The vertebral and basilar arteries give branches to the medulla, pons, and cerebellum, supplying these structures with most of their blood supply.

Near the top of the pons the carotid arteries and the basilar artery send branches to each other. These branches form a complete circle, called the Circle of Willis after the anatomist who discovered it. If any one artery becomes blocked on its way to the brain, blood from the other arteries can flow into it at the Circle of Willis, providing some circulation to the parts of the brain it would normally serve. The system is not perfect, however, and the Circle of Willis may not always provide enough blood flow to prevent a stroke if one artery is obstructed.

From the Circle of Willis, several large arteries provide blood flow to different areas of the brain. Since there are no branches connecting

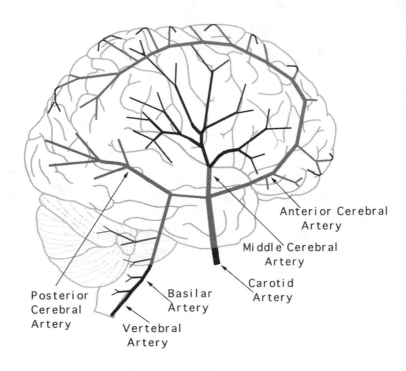

Figure 2.1   The major arteries of the brain.

these arteries to each other, obstruction of any one of them will always result in a stroke. If a very large artery becomes blocked, large areas of the brain are affected and the stroke is severe. If only a small branch is blocked, a small stroke results, but complete recovery is possible if other parts of the brain can take over the function of that area.

There are three large arteries that provide blood to the cerebral hemisphere on each side. These are, in order, the Anterior, Middle, and Posterior Cerebral Arteries, which supply blood to the front, middle, and back of the cerebrum (Fig. 2.1). The posterior cerebral artery also supplies blood to the temporal lobe and part of the cerebellum. Knowing the anatomy of the arteries, it's fairly simple to know which part of the brain will be affected by a stroke involving

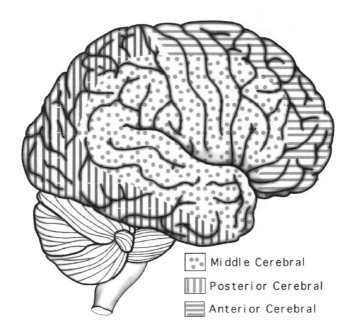

Middle Cerebral

Posterior Cerebral

Anterior Cerebral

Figure 2.2   The areas of the cerebral cortex supplied by each of the three cerebral arteries. *By comparing this to Fig. 1.6, you can see the types of brain functions that would be affected by a stroke involving any one of the cerebral arteries.*

that artery (Fig. 2.2). By comparing Fig. 2.2 with Fig. 1.6, it becomes apparent what type of functions can be lost to strokes involving each artery.

A stroke involving the middle cerebral artery often causes paralysis and loss of sensation in the face and arm because these areas of the brain are supplied by this artery. Strokes of the posterior cerebral artery may cause blindness, inability to understand speech (if Wernicke's area is affected), or problems with emotions, memory, and sensory processing. Strokes of the anterior cerebral artery often cause abnormal behaviors and thought patterns and may also cause paralysis of the leg.

Strokes involving the basilar artery's smaller branches affect the brain stem and cerebellum. As mentioned in chapter 1, the brain stem contains many densely packed tracts transmitting messages between the brain and the body. It also contains parts of the brain that control consciousness, breathing, blood pressure regulation, and a host of other functions. For this reason, strokes in the basilar artery system can cause severe and often unpredictable problems.

Given today's technology, it is possible to remove and correct problems in the carotid arteries. This prevents thousands of strokes each year. Unfortunately, it is currently not possible to correct problems in the vertebral and basilar arteries, or in the arteries inside the skull. When vascular disease occurs in these areas, medications may reduce the risk of stroke, but it is not possible to correct or remove existing obstructions.

Although the most frequent neurologic problem involving blood vessels is a stroke—lack of blood flow to part of the brain—blood vessel abnormalities can cause other problems. The most common is hemorrhage (bleeding). Hemorrhage obviously occurs if the blood vessels are cut, which can happen if a sharp bone fragment from a skull fracture pierces the wall of a blood vessel. In some people, especially older people, the blood vessels may be stretched and torn by a head injury that doesn't result in a skull fracture.

Another source of bleeding is a ruptured aneurysm. An aneurysm is a weakening of the wall of a blood vessel that forms a balloonlike outpouching. Aneurysms can occur in any part of the body, but those near the brain are referred to as cerebral aneurysms. If the weakening is severe enough, or if blood pressure rises high enough, the balloon bursts and bleeding into or on the surface of the brain occurs. The first symptom of a ruptured aneurysm is often an incredibly severe, sudden headache. Loss of consciousness may follow within minutes to a few hours. If an aneurysm is discovered before it ruptures completely, it can be repaired by surgery.

Aneurysms and trauma usually cause bleeding on the brain's surface. The most common cause of bleeding inside the brain itself is high blood pressure. The small arteries in the brain have very thin walls. If the blood pressure becomes very high, the thin walls may rupture, resulting in bleeding inside the brain tissue. Because this blood is under very high pressure, it can tear through the brain tissue and destroy neurons and tracts of fibers.

Medically, when bleeding occurs inside the skull but outside the brain, it is referred to as either a subdural (under the dural membranes) or epidural (outside the dural membranes but within the skull) hemorrhage. While this bleeding is not actually inside the brain, the collection of blood within the skull can crush brain tissue and cause permanent damage. When bleeding occurs within the brain, it is referred to as an intracerebral (intra means within, cerebral means brain) hemorrhage. This type of bleeding always results in permanent damage to some degree.

The Blood–Brain Barrier

One aspect of the brain's blood vessels is so different from blood vessels in other parts of the body—and so important in many ways—that it deserves special mention. In most parts of the body, any small molecules in the blood can pass freely through the walls of blood vessels and into tissues. This is, of course, how oxygen and nutrients get into tissues. It is also the way that drugs and toxins reach the same locations.

The brain's blood vessels do not let substances pass into brain tissues nearly as easily as do vessels in other parts of the body. Oxygen and nutrients pass freely enough, but many drugs are unable to pass through the blood–brain barrier. Some antibiotics and chemotherapy, for example, are not useful in treating brain diseases because the molecules of medication cannot pass through the blood–brain barrier.

Interestingly, when the brain is damaged or swollen, the blood–brain barrier often stops working. It is possible to take advantage of this in some cases. For example, an antibiotic that normally would not pass into the brain may indeed be able to if the brain is irritated by an infection. When this is the case, the antibiotic will reach parts of the brain that are infected and swollen, even though it does not reach the parts that aren't infected.

CHAPTER 3

How the Brain Functions

No one really understands how the brain accomplishes everything that it does. There is a lot of speculation about how the brain actually works: What is consciousness? How do we think? How do we remember? Scientists argue and discuss these topics endlessly, but there are no clear-cut answers at this time.

What scientists have been able to do, however, is to find the exact areas of the brain that perform certain specific functions and learn a little bit about how these areas interact. Some of this knowledge, particularly concerning the functions of different parts of the cerebral cortex, has been available for more than a century. The first evidence that certain parts of the brain had specific functions was obtained by simple observation. A patient would have an injury to one area of the brain and doctors would note what functions were lost due to that injury.

The most famous example of this was the report of Phineas Gage, a railroad worker whose skull was pierced by a metal rod in 1848. Gage survived even though the frontal lobes of his brain were damaged. He moved and talked without difficulty, his memory was fine, and his intellect appeared unaltered. After the injury, however, he changed from a cheerful, sensible, and popular man to a bad tempered drinker, notable for being incredibly stubborn and profane. This was the first evidence that the brain's frontal lobes were involved in regulating emotion and behavior.

Beginning in 1861, Paul Broca (for whom Broca's area of the brain is named) performed autopsies on the brains of stroke victims. He compared the functions a person was known to have lost following a stroke to areas of brain damage he found at autopsy. From this he was able to determine the functions of particular brain regions. Broca's work developed the first general maps delineating the function of the cerebral cortex's various areas. By the late 1800s, doctors knew the general function of each part of the cerebral cortex.

Later, when it became possible to operate on the brain, surgery was often performed using local anesthesia. After removing a piece of the skull to expose the brain, doctors would stimulate the brain as they operated. (The brain itself has no pain sensation, so patients were quite comfortable while this was being done). Stimulating a certain area might cause a finger to move, while stimulating another area would cause the patient to hear a sound. In this way, more accurate brain maps were made, indicating what specific functions almost every square inch of the cerebral cortex had. Since the brain's deeper structures couldn't be reached by this method, the functions of these areas remained mostly unknown.

Today, particularly since PET scans (see chapter 4) have been developed, scientists can literally watch the brain function while people perform complex tasks, such as solving mathematical problems or speaking. Over the last ten years, we have actually seen how the brain's various areas connect and interact with each other.

These kinds of studies have allowed much more specific maps of the brain's functions to be made and have begun to show us how the brain actually works. For example, PET scan studies have shown that when a person is asked to name animals, an area of the left medial occipital lobe (a part of the brain involved in visual processing) is activated. Naming tools activates an area in the left middle temporal gyrus—the area involved in hand movements. Naming objects of either type activates the part of the temporal lobe used to form speech. In other words, naming certain types of objects always activates the part of the temporal lobe we've long known was the speech center, but it also activates secondary areas of the brain; the secondary areas activated depend upon the properties of the object being thought of.

We've also learned that while the brain is organized in separate modules for different functions, the modules are flexible rather than rigid—its organization can change to some degree over time. We now know that the brain remodels itself constantly, forming new connections among neurons as they absorb new experiences and create new memories. When a basketball player practices thousands of shots, his brain actually makes new connections that allow his hands and eyes to coordinate better. Similarly, a stroke patient can relearn how to walk as new areas of the brain become involved in making the muscles of the legs work. Obviously, there are limits to how much remodelling the brain can do, however.

It's not surprising that the 1990s have been declared "The Decade of the Brain." Most neuroscientists agree that more has been learned about the brain in the last twenty years than in all history. It must be emphasized, however, that even this knowledge can only show us how the brain functions to perform very simple tasks. We cannot even begin to find a "thinking" area of the brain, much less a "golf swing" area of the brain.

Specific Functions of the Cerebral Cortex

No matter which part of the cerebral cortex is examined, the overall structure is similar (see Fig. 1.2 on page 9). The outer layer (the gray matter) is composed of individual neuron's (nerve cells) cell bodies. The inner layer (the white matter) consists of long axons (the strands that transmit the nerve's electrical signals) projected from the cell bodies in the gray matter. From any part of the cortex some axons pass from one area to another within the same hemisphere. Other axons pass from one hemisphere to the other through the large structure called the corpus callosum that connects the two hemispheres. Still other axons descend from the cortex to other parts of the brain and finally to the spinal cord.

Although the cerebral cortex looks very similar in appearance anywhere on the surface of the brain, each area of the cortex is involved in a single very specific function. While no two people will have exactly the same appearance of the gyri and sulci (the peaks and valleys of the cortex), everyone's brain is so similar that a general map showing the function of each brain area will be accurate to within a fraction of an inch for a given person.

Although the cortex is perhaps the most complex processing area of the brain, and is certainly the part of the brain that is understood best, it does not work alone. For example, the impulse to pick your right foot off the floor originates in the motor cortex. When the impulse leaves the cortex, it passes to the cerebellum and several nuclei (areas of cells deep within the brain) that automatically send unconscious signals to various muscles so that you transfer your weight to the other foot, tense muscles in the trunk to maintain your balance, etc. Without input from these brain areas you could still lift your right foot off the floor but you would probably fall over every time you tried.

THE DOMINANT AND NONDOMINANT HEMISPHERES

The two halves of the cerebral cortex (right and left) each control the opposite side of the body, and to a large extent are mirror images of each other. For example, the motor area for the right side of your body (on the left cortex) is an exact replica of the motor area for your left side (on the right cortex). A few areas of the cortex function differently on either side, however. Some of these functions are handled only by the dominant hemisphere (the left side of the brain in over 90 percent of people), while others are performed only by the nondominant hemisphere. In popular psychology, these are referred to as "left brain" and "right brain" functions.

For example, only the dominant hemisphere contains the areas necessary to understand and create speech, writing, and other forms of verbal communication. It also appears to contain the primary areas that perform mathematical calculations, such as addition and multiplication. The nondominant hemisphere contains the areas that recognize and process spatial constructions (geometric patterns, judging size and distance, and others), as well as areas that recognize emotion and process musical patterns and songs.

The two halves of the brain communicate with each other via the corpus callosum, a thick band of fibers travelling between the right and left hemispheres. In a few rare forms of epilepsy and other diseases, surgeons must cut the corpus callosum to prevent seizures from spreading. Experiments on these "split-brain" patients appear to indicate that each half of the brain has a mind or consciousness of its own. Since the dominant hemisphere controls speech, however, only it can communicate to the outside world.

For example, if the left hand (controlled by the right hemisphere) of a split-brain subject touches an object that the person can't see, the right hemisphere becomes aware of it. Later, if asked, the person can point to the object they touched with their left hand, but not their right hand. If the person is asked to say what object they touched, the person will truthfully say that they do not know, since the left hemisphere (which controls speech) received no information about what the left hand has touched.

THE FRONTAL LOBES

The primary motor cortex is located in the precentral gyrus (see Fig. 1.2 on page 9), which is considered the start of the frontal lobe in each cortex. The primary motor cortex actually processes and sends the movement impulse to the part of the body involved. The area just in front of the primary motor cortex is concerned with the initiation (or idea) of the particular movement, deciding what muscles should move to perform the actual task the person wants to accomplish.

The prefrontal cortex (the very front of the frontal lobes, not including the motor cortex) is concerned with higher intellectual functions and behavior. This is the area of higher brain function that inhibits certain primitive behaviors, such as rage. Destruction of this area results in a loss of concentration and a lack of judgment.

THE PARIETAL LOBES

The parietal lobe is concerned primarily with interpreting and understanding the body's sensory inputs. The primary sensory cortex is located in the postcentral gyrus (Fig. 1.2), which is considered the most forward part of the parietal lobe. The primary sensory cortex is the part of the brain that perceives the sensations of touch, vibration, and the position sense of the body (knowing that your knee is bent, for example). Destruction of this area results in partial or complete loss of some (or all) sensations in some part of the body.

The remainder of the parietal lobe is generally concerned with integrating (putting several sensations together to form a mental image or bit of knowledge). Integration is what happens when you pet something warm and soft, hear purring, and automatically think "cat." Destruction of the parietal lobe can cause clumsiness, inability to interpret spatial relationships, and an inability to integrate multiple sensory inputs into a single mental picture.

THE OCCIPITAL LOBES

The occipital lobes contain the visual cortex, the area of the brain that "sees." Damage to this area on one side of the brain may produce a loss of vision on the opposite side of the body (for example, although both eyes function, the person cannot see anything to their right side). Damage in other parts of the occipital lobe may result in a lack of ability to interpret vision. For example, a person may see a car, but be unable to judge what direction the car is moving in, or how rapidly it is moving.

Research in 1998 at the National Institute of Mental Health suggests that the abnormalities of the visual cortex are present in people with dyslexia. Apparently, dyslexic men are less able to detect visual motion than nondyslexic men. Additionally, an area of the brain known as V5, located at the junction of the occipital and temporal lobes, is less active in dyslexic people than others. This area aids in determining the direction of movement, and perhaps is important in determining the correct order of letters to form a word.

THE TEMPORAL LOBES

The posterior part of the temporal lobe (the part nearest the parietal and occipital lobes) is known as the auditory cortex. It receives and interprets sound information, and on the dominant hemisphere contains the area that understands speech. The inner part of the temporal lobe (near the brain stem) is the olfactory cortex, which is concerned with the sense of smell. The front of the temporal lobe is involved in emotions and works with the frontal lobe and other areas of the brain involved in emotion. Inside the cortex near the tip of the temporal lobe is a large nuclei of cells known as the amygdala, which appears to be an area that stores and processes emotional memories.

Some particularly interesting research in Germany suggests that an area in the temporal lobe in the dominant hemisphere is much larger in musicians compared to nonmusical people and is even larger in musicians who have "perfect pitch." This area of the brain develops at around the thirtieth week of pregnancy, giving some credence to those who claim playing music to a baby in the womb can affect later musical ability. It is particularly surprising that this area is located in the dominant hemisphere because most of the brain's music processing areas are located in the nondominant hemisphere.

The Cerebellum

The cerebellum, which looks like a wrinkled ball fitting just behind and under the cerebral cortex, is primarily associated with coordinating and managing movement, maintaining balance and posture, and similar functions. Recent studies suggest that the cerebellum also processes some sensory information involving concepts, such as the texture and shape of objects.

The Midbrain and Brain Stem

The largest portion of the midbrain is the thalamus. This area seems to be the main relay station connecting the cerebral cortex to the rest of the brain and body. Some processing occurs at the thalamus, and it may be that the thalamus actually "decides" which sensory information actually reaches the cerebral cortex. For example, you are not consciously aware of the touch of clothes on your body even though sensory input is always arriving to the brain. The thalamus apparently decides which information is important enough for you to become consciously aware of.

The hypothalamus, located just in front of the thalamus, is the area concerned with regulating body functions. It controls body temperature and is where appetite originates. The hypothalamus is attached directly to the pituitary gland, which controls the levels of various hormones that regulate bodily functions.

New Advances in Understanding How the Brain Works

Most of the topics discussed in the following section describe areas of new discoveries. As further research is done, the conclusions involving these subjects may change a little or a lot. Even though these individual facts may change as we gain further understanding of the brain and its function, it's interesting to learn how the brain may actually work. More importantly, these new ideas about how the brain functions help us to understand why certain types of brain disease or damage may have certain effects.

Most of the studies in this field use computed tomography (CT) and magnetic resonance imaging (MRI) to evaluate the brain's structure. Single-photon emission computed tomography (SPECT) and positron emission tomography (PET) are used to evaluate brain function. These tests are discussed in further detail in chapter 4.

EMOTIONS AND EMOTIONAL MEMORY

It has long been known that the frontal lobes, along with the amygdala (an area inside the temporal lobe) and the hippocampus (a small area deep within the brain located near the thalamus), are involved with emotion. Recent studies have indicated that "emotional memory" is different than normal memory for facts and past events (called "declarative memory"). Apparently, emotional memory involves different areas of the brain compared to declarative memory—namely the amygdala.

MRI and PET scans are providing evidence that severe emotional trauma actually changes the brain's structure and decreases the size of certain parts of the hippocampus. Victims of severe childhood sexual abuse and veterans who have suffered combat-related posttraumatic stress disorder have smaller hippocampal areas than other people.

These areas are essential for transfer of short-term memories into permanent storage, so it isn't surprising that people with posttraumatic stress disorder tend to have problems with their short-term memory.

REASONING AND THOUGHT

PET scans have shown that simple tests of reasoning activate only the prefrontal cortex, while more complex reasoning and problem-solving activate both these areas and the hippocampus. It is likely that the hippocampus becomes active as the brain searches for memories that can find a solution to the problem.

One interesting outcome of research into thought processes has been studies of the brains of psychotherapy patients. Researchers at the University of California at Los Angeles reported that ten weeks of psychotherapy not only improved the symptoms of six people with obsessive-compulsive disorder, but that PET scans indicated that four brain areas whose functions had been tightly linked in the patients before therapy had loosened and worked independently of one another after therapy. The effects were similar to those observed after treating the disorder with tranquilizers or antidepressant medications.

Another experiment at Harvard University seems to show how the brain determines if a memory is actually true. Those conducting the experiment read lists of words to twelve women. Ten minutes later the researchers read somewhat different lists and asked which words on the second list were not on the first list. PET scans performed during the experiment revealed that the hippocampus (the center for memory retrieval) lit up whether the women were recalling either a word that they had actually heard or one that they only thought they heard. When recalling words that they actually had heard, however, the scan also showed activation in the left temporal parietal area (where sounds are decoded). The true memory had apparently retrieved not just the word but also the actual sound of the word. When a subject recalled a word erroneously only the hippocampus lit up.

MEMORY

One of the more surprising findings in brain research has been that there is no one area of the brain devoted to memory. Rather there are central regions of the brain that act as directors or relayers of memory, while the actual individual memories are stored at various locations. In one study, scientists at the University of Pennsylvania Medical Center gave their study subjects two tasks to perform that involved memory: one was to identify vegetables on a list of miscellaneous words; the other was to specify which of two squares contained a dot in the same location as a target square.

A special type of MRI revealed activation in the left temporal lobe (the language center) for the word list task and in the parietal-occipital region (the spacial reconstruction area) for the dot location task. With either task the prefrontal cortex and the cingulate gyrus (an area in the center of the brain that is connected to the prefrontal cortex) became active. It is postulated that perhaps these latter areas bring stored information into conscious thought.

RESEARCH ON NEUROLOGIC AND PSYCHIATRIC DISEASES

Neurodegenerative diseases such as Alzheimer's disease, disorders such as alcoholism, and even the normal aging process can severely impair a person's ability to think clearly or rationally. In many of these diseases, structural and physiological changes occur in the brain, presumably causing some or all of the symptoms. Advances in brain imaging techniques have allowed us to study these changes accurately and indicate how the changes cause certain symptoms.

Brain imaging research is also resulting in remarkable observations about a number of poorly understood brain dysfunctions, including some problems that historically have been considered purely psychiatric or psychological in nature. Active studies are revealing new information about schizophrenia, depression, obsessive-compulsive disorder, Tourette's syndrome, attention deficit disorder, Alzheimer's disease, and many others.

I'll mention a few such areas of research in this section because they are interesting and illustrate how even subtle problems with how the brain functions may cause significant illness. Please note that all the discussion in this section concerns new research that is not yet clearly understood. Though fascinating facts are being discovered about several of these diseases, it is far too early to draw any definite conclusions about them.

ALZHEIMER'S DISEASE AND SENILITY

In patients with Alzheimer's disease, SPECT and PET scans reveal that blood flow to the parietal lobes of the cerebral cortex is very low, a situation also present in other forms of dementia (severe disturbances of thought), and in Parkinson's disease. This altered blood flow is probably a symptom rather than a cause of the problem, however. Other studies suggest that in Alzheimer's disease the brain either produces less of certain cell proteins, or the proteins are breaking down too rapidly. The studies do indicate that Alzheimer's disease is clearly different than senility (dementia occurring in older age, often the result of multiple small strokes or other processes that damage brain cells).

SCHIZOPHRENIA

Schizophrenia has been studied more extensively than any other psychiatric disorder. MRI and CT scans show that the ventricles (fluid-filled interior cavities of the brain) are larger than normal in the brains of schizophrenic patients, as are the surface grooves of the brain's surface. Most studies also suggest that schizophrenic patients have reduced tissue in the temporal lobes of the cerebral cortex and in the limbic region, which regulates emotion and memory. Most of these abnormalities apparently existed before schizophrenic symptoms develop.

Other studies also show abnormalities in the frontal lobes and thalamus of schizophrenic patients. People who are not schizophrenic but suffer brain damage in this region sometimes develop symptoms associated with schizophrenia, which include apathy, emotional unresponsiveness, and social withdrawal.

Some PET studies suggest that in addition to tissue loss in the frontal lobes, schizophrenic patients also have low metabolic activity in these areas. In normal people, two standard experimental tasks that produce high blood flow in that region are the Continuous Performance Test, which requires sustained attention, and the Wisconsin Card Sort Test, which requires the capacity to change one's mind in response to new information. Prefrontal blood flow increases relatively little in schizophrenic patients when they take these tests.

These findings suggest that schizophrenia may result from a breakdown in connections between the frontal lobes and the rest of the brain. Many researchers believe that in schizophrenic patients a brain injury or malfunction affecting the prefrontal cortex is present at birth and lies dormant until adolescence. During hormonal changes that occur at adolescence, the defect in connections between the frontal and temporal lobes and the limbic system becomes symptomatic.

DEPRESSION

PET scans suggest that happiness reduces brain activity in some areas while sadness increases it in others. Happiness is associated with lower blood flow (and therefore lower activity) in the prefrontal region and the temporal-parietal area. The prefrontal region of the dominant hemisphere has increased activity during ordinary sadness (though not in people with clinical depression). The amygdala, a part of the limbic system that regulates memory for emotionally significant events, is more active than normal in clinical depression. This pattern is also apparent in patients who may not be clinically depressed at present but have been in the past. Recent highly detailed MRI scans show that the hippocampus, another part of the limbic system, is smaller than average in people with a history of depression and that the longer a person has been depressed, the smaller his or her hippocampus will be.

OTHERS

People with severe obsessive-compulsive disorder have pointless but irresistible thoughts and perform repetitive actions. In mild cases, this may mean compulsive neatness or an inability to stop a "nervous habit." In severe cases, people can become incapacitated and unable to function because they constantly perform repetitive rituals. PET and fMRI (functional magnetic resonance imaging) scans of obsessive-compulsive patients taken while their symptoms are active (when a person with a germ obsession holds a dirty towel, for example) indicate abnormal activity in certain parts of the frontal cortex. MRI images suggest a loss of tissue in the caudate nucleus, an area of neurons located deep within the cerebral cortex.

Apparently the caudate is not performing its normal function of preventing vagrant thoughts from being translated into action. The circuit that includes the caudate, areas of the frontal cortex, and the thalamus is hyperactive because the feedback mechanisms that should quiet it down are not working. As a result, obsessional thinking (registered on PET scans as high frontal activity) persists until a compulsive ritual stops it. As mentioned earlier, recent experiments suggest that this pattern changes after successful treatment with either drugs or psychotherapy. PET scans then show less energy consumption in the caudate, apparently because the self-sustaining circuit of obsessional thoughts and compulsive behavior has been broken.

Attention deficit disorder (ADD) occurs most commonly in male children while affecting females and adults only occasionally. Characteristic symptoms include hyperactivity, being easily distracted, and impulsiveness. Imaging studies of children with ADD reveal several abnormalities, although precisely what they mean is not yet clear. In one study, CT scans found boys with ADD had less tissue in the corpus callosum, the band joining the two hemispheres of the cerebral cortex, than boys without ADD. Another found that ADD children had a smaller right frontal lobe and an enlarged caudate nucleus in the left hemisphere. PET scans indicated lower-than-average activity in these same regions during experimental tasks that demand a person's concentration. Treatment with stimulant drugs, which help ADD children to concentrate, temporarily eliminates this latter irregularity.

Imaging scans also reveal that the brains of men and women are much more different than had ever been suspected (scientists certainly didn't expect it). For example, while it has long been known that the brain loses volume as it ages, MRIs have shown that the patterns of loss differ in men and women. Men tend to lose volume all over the brain with most of the loss occurring in the frontal and temporal lobes. Women tend to lose more volume from the hippocampus and parietal lobes.

Other studies have shown that when men speak, only the major speech areas of the dominant hemisphere of the brain become active. When women speak, several other areas of the brain also become involved. Clinically, doctors have known for years that women have an easier time recovering from strokes that affected their speech. It may be that these "accessory" speech areas are increasingly able to compensate if major speech areas are damaged.

CHAPTER 4

Medical Tests of the Brain and Brain Function

During the last two decades a virtual explosion of medical technology has allowed us to examine the brain in more depth and detail than a physician in the 1960s would have ever dreamed possible. Multimillion dollar equipment can "see" inside the skull, showing us the anatomy of the brain in incredible detail. Some types of scans can actually "watch" the brain at work—observing which areas of the brain become active during certain tasks. Other tests can evaluate the tiny electrical currents generated as messages travel to and fro in the brain, and laboratory analysis can determine the chemical composition of fluids that bathe the brain.

The fact that diagnostic tests for neurologic disease are very good understandably leads many people to think they are perfect. The reality, however, is far different. Each of these tests has its strengths, weaknesses, and risks. It has also been argued that it is now easier for a doctor to order a lot of tests rather than carefully examine the patient to determine which tests are really necessary. And in these days of managed health care, it must be mentioned that almost all these tests are quite expensive. In some cases the insurer will not pay for a certain test unless specific circumstances exist. For all these reasons, it is important that any person being evaluated for neurologic disease have a good understanding of what each test involves, what information it may provide to the doctor, and what it cannot determine.

The Physician's Examination

Given today's high-tech electronic diagnosis capability, many people do not realize that the best diagnostic test is a careful evaluation performed by an experienced physician. Even some physicians forget this fact, ordering $1,000 tests without taking the time to determine if they are truly necessary.

Physicians experienced in evaluating and treating neurologic disease possess an incredible amount of knowledge about the nervous system's anatomy and function. By carefully determining the areas of brain function that aren't working properly, a good neurologist or neurosurgeon can usually tell exactly where (to within fractions of an inch) a problem in the brain is located. They will then know what test is most likely to reveal precisely what disease is causing the problem.

Some patients become frustrated or irritated by a neurologic examination. It can take over an hour of carefully testing muscle strength, reflexes, sensations, and even thought processes to complete. If you've had such an examination, you may have thought to yourself, "Why don't they just do a CT scan and see what's wrong?"

The reality is that the examination may actually be more accurate than the scan. Even if it's not, the information obtained during a neurologic examination narrows down the area to be tested and tells the doctor what type of problem he should concentrate on when he orders and evaluates the tests. Perhaps more importantly, it tells the doctor what tests are not necessary, thus avoiding potential complications and unnecessary expense.

WHAT'S THE DIFFERENCE BETWEEN NEUROLOGISTS AND NEUROSURGEONS?

The obvious difference between a neurologist and a neurosurgeon, of course, is that only the neurosurgeon performs operations. Some people, therefore, think of the neurosurgeon as a "better" doctor, or one who can do everything. In reality, the two often work together to make a diagnosis. Depending upon the actual condition involved, one or the other will be more qualified to treat the patient.

Neurosurgeons spend six or more years after residency in specialty training. Obviously, one focus of their training is learning how to perform operations and care for patients before and after surgery, but much of their training involves how to diagnose neurologic conditions that may require surgery, such as brain tumors or aneurysms. Neurologists spend four to six years in training after medical school. Like neurosurgeons, the majority of their training involves the diagnosis of neurological disease, but they also focus on treating neurological problems with medication, rehabilitation, and other therapies. Most neurologists are also trained in internal medicine or psychiatry.

PATIENT HISTORY AND PHYSICAL EXAMINATION

The purpose of a patient history is to provide the doctor with enough information so that he can make a differential diagnosis, that is, a list of several conditions that are most likely causing the patient's symptoms. The question-and-answer process involved can be a bit time consuming, but dozens of medical studies have shown it constitutes the most important part of determining what condition or disease the patient is suffering from. In fact, for problems involving headache, dizziness, memory loss, or difficulty in thinking properly, a patient history is more likely to provide the correct diagnosis than all other tests combined.

As a patient, the most important thing you can do to expedite the process is to provide accurate and complete information about your medical history and symptoms. Nothing is more important than providing complete information about your past medical history and the history of your present problem. Writing things down before you go to the doctor's office is often invaluable. At the very least, make a list of all your medications, allergies, and medical conditions. Most doctors will not even begin to consider ordering tests until they have this information.

A second aid to a patient history is being able to describe all symptoms accurately in plain everyday terms. "I'm having migraine headaches" provides very little information for the doctor to assess. "I'm having headaches starting behind my right ear and running to my forehead, usually starting in the afternoon" provides a whole lot more information. Areas of the body that are numb, seem weak or uncoordinated, have pain, or sometimes tremble should be mentioned. Any difficulties in performing everyday tasks can provide important clues, as can changes in mood or memory.

Two other symptoms can be difficult to describe but can provide invaluable information to the doctor: the description of pain and the description of the time course of the problem. Pain, in particular, is difficult to describe (bad, really bad, or horrible doesn't help the evaluation very much). If your condition involves pain, you might look at some of the following words that neurologists commonly use to describe pain to see which ones describe the type of pain you experience. Notice that for purposes of diagnosing a condition the characteristics of the pain are more important than its severity.

- Aching
- Throbbing
- Cramping
- Gnawing
- Burning
- Heavy
- Tingling
- Itching
- Shooting
- Stabbing
- Dull
- Sharp
- Tender
- Splitting

- Nauseating
- Flickering
- Hypersensitive

The time course of the problem should be described in two ways. The first part of the time course is how the condition has progressed since it started. For example, an occasional pain in one part of the body that spread over a few months to become more severe and involve other parts of the body is quite different from a pain that started suddenly one morning and never changed. The second part of the time course involves variations from day-to-day or within each day. Pain may be constant, it may be worse in the evening or morning, or it may change at random. It may also be worse during certain activities or in certain positions.

There is not much you can do to help the doctor with the physical examination other than cooperating. A neurologic physical examination always involves tests of muscle strength (usually comparing one side against the other), reflexes, coordination, and sensation. In general, all you are asked to do is perform a series of simple tasks, such as walking with your eyes closed, balancing on one foot or the other, touching a moving object, and reporting whether you feel light touches or pinpricks on various parts of your body.

The purpose of these procedures is to determine what parts of the nervous system may not be working properly. Several different parts of the nervous system are involved in most functions. For example, if you're having trouble touching your right index finger to a moving object, the problem could involve either the part of the brain that processes vision, the motor area of the brain that controls the hand and arm, the cerebellum controlling arm coordination, the fiber tracts in the brain connecting all these areas, or the fiber tracts leaving the brain to control the nerves of the arm. By performing several other tests involving each of these different areas, the doctor can usually narrow the problem down to just one specific part of the brain.

Patients are often surprised by the amount of time their physician will spend examining their eyes. More than any other part of the body, the eyes provide a "window" into the brain: the eyes receive nerve endings from four of the twelve cranial nerves, and their blood supply is closely interconnected to that of the brain.

It is important that you not exaggerate your symptoms during the physical examination—which some people tend to do to make sure the doctor fully realizes that they really have something wrong with them. What usually happens when a patient exaggerates symptoms is that the doctor tends not to believe them because their symptoms don't follow any known neurologic patterns.

For example, several neurologic conditions cause the outside, back part of one hand to be numb (the area of the ring finger and little finger) below the wrist. The most common condition that makes the entire hand numb from the wrist down is malingering (faking an illness). A patient who tells the doctor their whole hand is numb is usually surprised when the doctor isn't very impressed with the seriousness of their condition. Even if the doctor still believes the patient has a serious problem, it becomes impossible for them to narrow down what is causing the condition because they can't accurately determine what parts of the nervous system are involved.

ROUTINE OFFICE TESTS

In addition to a history and physical examination, you may be asked to give a blood sample, have an electrocardiogram, undergo other routine medical tests, or have a mental status examination. In most cases, routine tests are ordered to rule out certain medical conditions that can cause neurologic symptoms. Diabetes, thyroid disease, certain infections, and rheumatoid arthritis all commonly cause neurologic problems, as do many other medical conditions.

The purpose of these tests is to make certain the neurologist or neurosurgeon isn't missing a basic medical condition that could be causing your symptoms. The doctor usually will expect these tests to come back normal or negative and may not mention them again. If any of them show that another disease may be present, you will usually be referred elsewhere to have that disease treated while the other neurologic tests are completed. In some cases, treatment of the underlying disease will be expected to clear up all the neurologic symptoms, meaning that no other diagnostic tests may be ordered until the underlying disease has been completely treated.

Some people are a bit anxious about taking a mental status examination, often because they think it is a "psychology" test or are afraid that the test results may be used to limit them from participating in certain activities. The mental status examination is actually the most sensitive test available for detecting certain types of problems in the brain. If detected, there are often fairly simple ways to retrain the affected person to overcome such problems. Obviously, if they are not detected, no treatment can be undertaken.

In most of these cases, the anatomy of the brain itself would appear normal to any type of scan or x-ray. However, there can still be significant problems with how the brain is functioning. Depending upon the type of problem the doctor suspects, the mental status examination may be nothing more than a simple test of memory or it may consist of a complex set of tests examining the way a person can process words or visualize three-dimensional items in space. A complex mental status examination can take half a day or so to administer.

X-Ray, CT Scan, and MRI Examinations

Three noninvasive types of tests are commonly used to help "see" the actual anatomy of the nervous system. The tests are referred to as noninvasive because they generally don't require any major procedures to be done to the patient. In general these tests have very low—almost no—chance of causing complications. They do expose the patient to either radiation (x-rays and CT scans) or a very strong magnetic field (MRI), but the risks resulting from x-ray exposure are negligible unless repeated many times. And from what we know currently, there are no risks from exposure to magnetic fields.

In some cases, a medication may be injected into a vein to enhance the test by making certain structures more visible. Whenever medication is injected, there is always the possibility of an allergic reaction, but the risk of this is fairly small.

STANDARD X-RAYS

Standard x-rays are almost never used in modern neurology. They can show the bones of the skull and spine, but provide almost no information regarding the brain or other parts of the nervous system. Even for a simple evaluation of the bones of the skull, other techniques, such as CT scans, provide much clearer images and are less likely to miss a fracture.

CT (COMPUTED TOMOGRAPHY) SCANS

CT scans use the same radiation as x-rays, but the x-ray tube is mounted inside a large doughnut-shaped device and moves around the patient in a circular fashion. Instead of exposing film like a standard x-ray, the radiation is detected by a series of sensors that feed information into a powerful computer. Because of the sensitivity of the sensors and the computer reconstruction, a CT scan can show the actual structures of the brain, blood vessels, and other tissues within the skull.

Each time the x-ray tube passes around the patient, it captures information from a narrow (about one-quarter-inch) cross section, referred to as a slice. Dozens of different slices are taken and printed together showing cross sections of the entire brain or area of the body being examined. Modern CT scans can demonstrate an abnormality less than half an inch in diameter.

Although a CT scan can tell the difference between bone, brain tissue, and some other types of tissue, it cannot always tell the difference between normal brain tissue, tumors, and other structures. In many cases a second CT scan will be done "with contrast." This involves injecting a liquid containing iodine or some other chemical that blocks x-rays into a vein and then repeats the CT scan. The contrast will absorb into any areas of the brain where the blood–brain barrier (see chapter 2) has been damaged and will show up as white areas on a CT scan. Contrast is often used to find small tumors or areas of the brain damaged by stroke. It can also be used to find an aneurysm (a balloonlike weakening of the wall) in the brain's blood vessels.

Having a CT scan is entirely painless, other than starting an IV if contrast will be needed. You will have to lie still while each slice is taken, but the entire process usually takes less than half an hour. The personnel performing the scan are in a separate room, but they can watch you through a window of leaded glass and can talk to you (and you can talk to them) through a microphone and speaker mounted in the scanner.

While the CT scan is an incredibly useful tool for studying the brain and spinal cord, it does have limitations. Parts of the brain stem and cerebellum are encased in such dense bone that the CT scan cannot show much detail about these parts of the brain. It also cannot detect some types of subtle changes in the brain itself. A "normal" CT scan doesn't mean that absolutely nothing is wrong, it simply means that there are no major abnormalities in the brain's structure.

There are few risks involved in a CT scan. Of course, you are exposed to x-ray radiation, and because of the number of images taken there is more exposure than occurs with standard x-rays. Even so, you could have many CT scans without any significant risk of problems from radiation. Pregnant women should not undergo a CT scan unless absolutely necessary, however, because the developing fetus is more sensitive to x-ray radiation than an adult.

If contrast media is injected, you could possibly have an allergic reaction that can sometimes prove severe. Contrast media also places some strain on your kidneys and can therefore cause problems in persons with kidney disease. Be certain to mention if you have any allergies to iodine, have ever had a reaction to x-ray contrast media, or have any kidney problems before you undergo a CT scan.

MRI (MAGNETIC RESONANCE IMAGING) SCANS

MRI scanners were developed long after CT scanners were in general use and are quite a bit more expensive and complicated than CT scanners. However, MRI scans have many advantages over CT scans and can show certain abnormalities of the brain that CT scans cannot detect. Like CT scans, the MRI requires a powerful computer to reconstruct its signals into a recognizable picture.

MRI scans do not use x-rays. Instead they use an extremely powerful magnetic field and radio waves to detect differences in the chemical structure of various tissues. The magnetic field in an MRI machine is as powerful as the electromagnets that junkyard operators use to pick up discarded cars. The magnetic force itself appears to be harmless to humans, but it is strong enough to ruin metal-containing objects, such as cardiac pacemakers, and electronic equipment located within a few feet of the machine.

An MRI scan does a much better job than a CT scan of showing the different tissues that comprise the brain, and it is particularly good at showing the difference between gray matter and white matter. MRI can also examine areas of the brain stem and cerebellum that are difficult to see on a CT scan. While MRI is often performed with the injection of contrast into a vein, the contrast used is not based on iodine, so it is less likely to affect the kidneys or cause an allergic reaction.

MRI can also show the brain's actual blood vessels, something a CT scan cannot do. In fact, an MRI scan can be used instead of arteriography (injection of dye into the arteries of the brain; see below) in many cases. When used for this purpose, MRI is often abbreviated to MRA, for Magnetic Resonance Arteriography. MRA cannot show the smaller arteries within the brain, however, so standard arteriography is still required in some cases.

Given all these advantages, it isn't surprising that MRI scans have become the test of choice to detect tumors, aneurysms and other blood vessel abnormalities, strokes, and brain injuries. It can even detect some types of diseases—multiple sclerosis, for example—that only change the character of brain tissue without altering the anatomy.

MRI has its shortcomings, however. Because of the strong magnetic fields used, persons who have certain metal devices—such as pacemakers—implanted in their bodies may not be able to have an MRI. It also can't evaluate the bones in the skull as well as a CT scan so it isn't as useful in examining people who've suffered head trauma.

Like CT scans, MRI scans are entirely painless unless you need an IV for injecting contrast dye. During the actual MRI, which takes about thirty minutes, you are placed in a closed tube, which some people have described as "coffin-like." You are able to talk to the people performing the test through a microphone but won't be able to see them. Very large people may have difficulty fitting inside the tube, and people with claustrophobia (fear of closed spaces) may not be able to tolerate being in a small enclosed area for the test. Most people tolerate the MRI quite well, however, and the doctor performing the test will usually give you a sedative or mild tranquilizer if you request one.

Two newer variations of MRI are used in certain special circumstances. Magnetic resonance spectroscopy (MRS) measures very small signals from several different types of atoms in the brain. MRS can measure the actual chemical makeup of the different tissues in the brain. For example, standard MRI can detect if a brain tumor is present but can't tell exactly what type of cancer is causing the tumor. MRS can distinguish between different types of brain tumors since each type has a slightly different chemical composition. The two disadvantages of MRS are its very high cost and that each slice of MRS requires minutes rather than mere seconds for a standard MRI.

Functional magnetic resonance imaging (fMRI) measures changes that occur when the level of blood oxygen rises in particular regions of the brain. The oxygen level reflects the amount of actual brain activity occurring in a specific region, so fMRI shows how hard a particular area of the brain is working. Currently, fMRI is being used in research to find out how the brain actually performs certain tasks, but in the future it will have added medical applications, such as providing guidance to brain surgeons.

Nuclear Medicine Scans

All nuclear medicine scans involve injecting a mildly radioactive medication into the bloodstream. Detectors outside the body determine exactly where the radioactive medication collects. Several different types of medications can be used, each of which is likely to collect in certain tissues. One, called spectamine, can be used to determine the blood flow to the brain and detect a stroke very early in its course. Other types can be used to detect infection in the brain or find certain types of tumors.

The amount of radiation you are exposed to in a nuclear medicine scan is minimal. The tests all are very low risk, although an allergic reaction to the medication is possible. In any case, these tests are not used very frequently.

PET and SPECT Scans

Positron emission tomography (PET) scans are similar to both nuclear medicine scans and CT scans. A medication is injected that releases positrons, a specific kind of radioactivity. The types of compounds that are used in PET scans tend to be involved in the metabolism of the brain and are particularly useful to show areas of the brain that are actively working. Where most scans show the anatomy of the brain, PET scans show how hard different areas of the brain are working.

For this reason, PET scans are used to "map" the brain, showing areas that have increased activity during tasks such as speaking or reading. Medically, PET scans can identify the location of areas involved in seizures, show if tumors are hyperactive (and therefore more likely to be malignant), or decide if the brain is functioning abnormally.

PET scans are very low-risk tests, but the equipment used is extremely expensive and isn't available in many areas. The radioactive medications used in PET scans have to be made just prior to use, requiring nuclear physicists and radiopharmacists to create the medication before each scan. Because most institutions lack such facilities, only a few hundred PET-scanning centers exist worldwide, most of them dedicated to research. While the equipment may become more widely available, it remains to be seen if the test will prove useful for many medical conditions.

Single photon emission computed tomography (SPECT) is a very long name for a test similar to a PET scan. Although SPECT images are not nearly as sharp and clear as PET scan images, the equipment and medications used are much simpler and less expensive. SPECT scans are sensitive enough to detect small abnormalities in the brain's chemical composition. For example, SPECT scans can determine the concentration of the chemical dopamine in various parts of the brain and detect abnormalities such as Parkinson's disease and Tourette's syndrome.

Lumbar Puncture (Spinal Tap) and Myelograms

Lumbar puncture simply means placing a needle between the bones of the lower back (the lumbar area) until it enters (or punctures) the sack containing cerebrospinal fluid. The procedure is fairly simple medically, and when performed properly, it causes only a little pain. The patient will usually be asked to curl into a ball while lying on their side, and after cleaning the lower back with iodine, the doctor will inject local anesthetic. After the area has become numb, a longer spinal needle is slipped between two of the bones of the back until it enters the sack of spinal fluid. Once the needle is in place, the doctor will ask you to lie still while he withdraws spinal fluid or takes other measurements.

Lumbar puncture has somewhat more risk than the other neurologic tests discussed above, but more than 99 percent of people who have the test experience absolutely no problems. Most people will have a mild backache for a day or two afterward. A few people, especially young women, will have a "spinal" headache after the procedure. This headache occurs only when the patient sits up and disappears when the patient lies down. In most cases, the headache will disappear after a couple of days, although the patient has to lie flat during that time.

It is not possible to damage the spinal cord by a lumbar puncture because the spinal cord ends at the middle of the back, above the level where the puncture is performed. However, the nerves to the legs do continue past the level of the lumbar puncture, and it is possible (although very rare) for the needle to scrape or irritate one of these nerves. Nerve irritation causes pain that emanates from the back and radiates down one leg. In most cases, the pain goes away completely in two to three weeks. Permanent nerve damage is extremely rare, occurring in less than one out of every one hundred thousand lumbar punctures.

A rare complication of lumbar puncture is infection at the puncture site. If you notice that the area where the puncture was performed becomes red and warm two or three days after the procedure, you should contact your doctor right away. Another rare complication is bleeding inside the backbone. For this reason, be certain to tell the doctor performing the procedure if you take any medication that prevents your blood from clotting, such as aspirin.

While there are some risks involved with a lumbar puncture, probably no single test can provide doctors with more information about the nervous system. The pressure of the spinal fluid can be measured to detect hydrocephalus or water on the brain. The cerebrospinal fluid can be analyzed to detect a number of chemical abnormalities, any type of infection, and some types of cancer.

Another test that requires a lumbar puncture is a myelogram. A myelogram is an x-ray taken after contrast medication has been injected into the spinal fluid. Myelograms are used to detect if any of the nerves in the spine are being pinched or compressed by a ruptured disc, bone spur, or tumor.

ARTERIOGRAPHY AND ULTRASONOGRAPHY

Arteriography, also called angiography, is an x-ray study that shows the arteries of the brain in great detail. It is used to detect obstruction in the large arteries bringing blood to the brain or to detect aneurysms and other abnormalities of the smaller arteries within the brain. Standard arteriography uses a catheter inserted into a large artery of the groin or arm and threaded through the aorta until it reaches the arteries near the brain. Dye is then injected and x-rays taken in a rapid series as the dye passes through the arteries in question.

The study itself is performed in a special x-ray room, with both heart and blood pressure monitored during the test. Most patients will be sedated for the test but will not be completely asleep. There is a little pain from the needle puncture into the artery in the groin, but the remainder of the test is fairly painless. Some people get a headache after the test, but it goes away in a few hours.

Arteriography has a higher complication rate than most of the other tests used in neurology. Possible complications include infection, bleeding at the injection site, a stroke, and having an allergic reaction. Overall, the complication rate of arteriography is still less than 0.5 percent, however.

An alternative to standard arteriography that can be used in many cases is digital subtraction arteriography. This technique uses computer enhancement of the x-rays so that dye can be injected into a vein in the arm rather than through a catheter threaded through the aorta. Digital subtraction arteriography has a lower complication rate than standard arteriography, but doesn't provide as clear a picture of the smaller arteries as standard arteriography does.

Ultrasound studies are performed by a machine that sends high frequency sound waves into the body, and then measures the waves as they are reflected back from the various structures in the area. Since the bones of the skull reflect these waves completely, ultrasound is not useful to examine the brain except during surgery. It is frequently used as a simple and safe test to detect disease in the carotid arteries, the large blood vessels found in the neck. The test itself is completely painless, requires no medication, and can usually be performed in fifteen to twenty minutes.

The Electroencephalogram (EEG)

The electroencephalogram (EEG) is commonly referred to as a "brain wave" test. The test has been in use since the early 1900s, and for most of the century was the only method available to examine how the brain functioned. Today the EEG is used mostly to evaluate people with epilepsy (seizures). It is also an important tool for assessing coma and other forms of brain damage.

The electrical waves detected by an electroencephalogram result from tiny electrical signals that the individual neurons in the brain create every time they send a signal. The overall current generated by the millions of neurons in any part of the brain is strong enough that it can be measured by electrodes placed over the surface of the scalp. Even so, the voltage involved is very small and requires special equipment to measure.

A standard EEG involves placing twenty-one electrodes in carefully measured positions over the scalp surface. The electrodes are attached with a paste, so no needle sticks are necessary. The procedure is entirely painless. There is no need to cut your hair before the procedure, but you will want to shampoo out the bits of paste that remain after the procedure is completed. For certain conditions, the EEG may also be measured during stimulations, such as shining a flashing light in front of your eyes. In a few cases, you will be asked to not sleep for a certain number of hours before the EEG, or the EEG may be taken while you are asleep.

A normal EEG recording is an unspectacular-looking chart, showing only the normal cyclic waves of brain activity measured at each electrode. Abnormally fast or slow cyclic waves can result from damage or disease of the entire brain, from the toxic effects of drugs, or from metabolic problems in the body.

The EEG of a person with epilepsy (seizures) will show characteristic large spikes of electrical activity, at least during a seizure. By examining each of the different electrodes, the neurologist can determine exactly what part of the brain initiates the seizure. This helps to determine which type of medication is most likely to stop the seizures, or can be used if surgery is needed to remove the epileptic focus (the damaged brain tissue that starts the seizure).

A variation of the EEG is the evoked potential. An evoked potential is the electrical activity that occurs in the brain in response to a stimulation. Since a specific stimulation only involves a small area of the brain and relatively few neurons, the electrical current generated is too small to measure directly. By repeating the stimulation many times, and using a computer specifically designed to amplify the response to that stimulation, the evoked potential can be measured, however.

Although it requires special equipment, having an evoked potential test is no different than undergoing an EEG—except for the stimulation involved. Three types of stimulation may be used. Visual evoked potentials record the response to altered light and darkness. Sensory evoked potentials record the response to electrical stimulation of a nerve near the wrist (and no, the stimulation is not painful). Auditory evoked potentials record the response to a clicking sound.

Electromyography (EMG) and Nerve Conduction Studies (NCS)

Electromyography (measurement of the electrical current in muscles) and nerve conduction studies (measurement of how well the body's nerves carry messages) are used primarily to study parts of the nervous system out in the body—not in the brain itself. They are most often used to diagnose damage to the nerves or spinal cord but can sometimes be used for other purposes.

In most cases, the entire test can be performed using electrodes applied to the skin with gel or paste. Occasionally it is necessary to insert a needle electrode under the skin to obtain an accurate reading, but this is unusual given today's modern equipment. In either test, a nonpainful (although strange feeling) electrical current is applied to the skin over a nerve, causing the nerve to transmit the current along its length. In electromyography, sensing electrodes measure the muscle's electrical response to that nerve signal. In nerve conduction studies, sensory electrodes measure how well the signal is transmitted along the nerve itself.

EMG and NCS can be used to evaluate muscular disease such as muscular dystrophy. They can determine the severity of nerve damage caused by trauma or diseases of the nervous system, or determine the location of injury to a nerve. They are commonly used to decide if a weakness is caused due to muscle disease, a peripheral nerve disease, or a problem in the brain or spinal cord.

PART II

Stroke and Vascular Disease of the Brain

CHAPTER 5

What Is a Stroke?

The simplest definition of stroke is the destruction of brain tissue caused by some malfunction of the brain's blood vessels. Medically, there are two major categories of stroke: ischemic and hemorrhagic. Ischemic stroke is by far the most common type of stroke; it is caused by the same type of vascular disease that causes heart attack. Ischemic means that there is not enough blood flow to an area, and therefore not enough oxygen to support the cells. When this occurs, the brain cells will first stop functioning, and then die if circulation is not restored quickly. Cell death caused by lack of blood flow is called infarction, so doctors will often refer to this type of stroke as a cerebral infarction.

Hemorrhage means bleeding, and a hemorrhagic stroke occurs when a blood vessel ruptures, causing bleeding inside the skull. Of course, hemorrhage can be caused by trauma, but hemorrhagic stroke is usually caused by hypertension (high blood pressure) or the rupture of an aneurysm, a balloonlike weakening of an artery's wall. No matter what the cause of hemorrhage, the bleeding can tear through the delicate connections within the brain and eventually compress brain cells to the point where they die.

Stroke is currently the third leading cause of disability and fifth leading cause of death in the United States. About 500,000 persons suffer a stroke each year, 150,000 of whom die from it. Stroke survivors may (or may not) be left with long-term problems depending on the severity of the stroke and its location in the brain.

The good news is that the majority of strokes are preventable, and new therapy is available to minimize the amount of damage that results when a stroke does occur. In order to understand how strokes are best prevented and treated, it is important to understand why they occur. This chapter will focus on what actually happens to the brain during a stroke rather than on the symptoms a person may experience during a stroke. The symptoms a person experiences during a stroke are discussed in more detail in chapter 7.

The Causes of Stroke

ATHEROSCLEROSIS AND VASCULAR DISEASE

Ischemic stroke almost usually results due to atherosclerosis, commonly known as hardening of the arteries. Atherosclerosis is caused by the deposit of fat into the walls of the arteries. The process begins as small streaks of fat are deposited just underneath the smooth lining of the arteries. As the disease progresses, the streaks become thick accumulations of fat, known as plaques. Eventually the plaques become large enough to project into the artery, causing partial obstruction of blood flow. Since the plaque's surface is rough and cracked, blood sometimes clots over the plaque, further obstructing the artery. Blood clotting within a blood vessel is known medically as thrombosis.

Atherosclerosis can, and does, occur in any artery of the body. One of the most common sites of atherosclerosis is in the coronary arteries supplying the heart, but it also frequently occurs in the arteries leading to the brain. When atherosclerosis occurs in these arteries, it is referred to as cerebral vascular disease.

When the obstruction becomes severe enough, blood flow to the part of the brain served by that artery decreases. If blood begins to clot over the plaque, blood flow can become totally obstructed causing a stroke. Alternatively, a piece of the plaque may break off in a large artery and be carried downstream until it blocks a smaller vessel (called embolism). In most cases, either thrombosis or embolism is the final event that completely occludes an artery and causes a stroke.

While we don't completely understand atherosclerosis, we do know of several risk factors, or behaviors and medical conditions, that make a person much more likely to develop the disease. Atherosclerosis is more likely to occur in males, smokers, people with high blood cholesterol levels or high blood pressure, and people who don't exercise frequently. While young women are unlikely to develop atherosclerosis, after menopause women are just as likely to develop the disease as are men.

Many (but not all) of these risk factors can be altered (see chapter 6), thus slowing the progress of the disease, or in some cases even reversing it. Additionally, there are medical and surgical therapies that can help prevent an actual stroke from occurring in a person who already has atherosclerosis. In order to decide which treatment is most likely to prove effective, doctors must first find the location of the atherosclerotic plaque. They must also determine if thrombosis or embolism is likely to play a role in a possible stroke.

The Arteries of the Brain

Exactly what symptoms a stroke will cause and how severe the stroke will be is determined primarily by which artery is involved. As discussed in chapter 2, there are four main arteries that carry blood to the brain: the two carotid arteries in the front of the neck (which carry most of the blood) and the two vertebral arteries that enter the brain along with the spinal cord at the base of the skull. As they enter the skull, the two vertebral arteries combine into a single artery called the basilar artery (see Fig. 2.1 on page 24).

Near the top of the brain stem, the basilar artery and the carotid arteries send branches, called communicating arteries, to each other. If an obstruction of any one of the major arteries occurs below the level of the communicating arteries, blood from the other arteries can flow through the communication, maintaining blood supply to areas of the brain served by the obstructed artery. If an obstruction occurs in any of the major branches higher than the communicating artery, there becomes no other avenue for blood flow to reach the affected area of the brain, and a stroke will occur.

Most strokes involve only one of the major blood vessels above the communicating artery: either the anterior cerebral, posterior cerebral, or middle cerebral arteries (see Fig. 2.1). Since these arteries are paired, one for each cerebral hemisphere, these strokes usually involve one side of the brain only. By comparing the illustrations in chapter 2, showing the areas of the brain served by each artery, with Fig. 1.6 (page 16), showing the function of the areas of each cerebral hemisphere, you can easily see what type of function would be affected by a stroke involving each artery. For example, a middle cerebral artery stroke would affect the ability to feel and move on one side of the body (since it affects one hemisphere), but would not greatly affect vision or the ability to hear.

Carotid Artery Disease

The carotid artery is commonly involved in atherosclerosis with plaques developing near the area where the artery branches, located at the upper part of the neck. Even if one of the carotids becomes completely obstructed, the other carotid and the basilar artery can often supply enough blood for the entire brain as long as the communicating arteries are intact.

If the carotid artery plaque becomes large and develops a rough surface, a piece of the plaque or a blood clot from the plaque can break off and travel up the carotid artery. This becomes an embolus when it lodges in a smaller branch of the carotid, causing a stroke to occur in the area served by that branch. Since it is uncommon for an embolus to pass through the communicating artery, this type of stroke usually involves a branch of the anterior cerebral or middle cerebral arteries, since these are the direct branches arising from the carotid artery.

A large embolus can obstruct either of the major branches or even the entire carotid artery resulting in a massive stroke. If the embolus is small (as is usually the case), only a small branch will be obstructed and the stroke will be limited to a small area of the brain. In some ways, a "warning stroke" such as this can prove lifesaving because it can alert the doctors to the presence of carotid artery disease. Surgery can then be performed to remove the plaque in the neck before a more massive stroke occurs.

Vertebrobasilar Artery Disease

Atherosclerosis in the vertebral and basilar artery can cause symptoms quite different than those for carotid disease. The main branches of the basilar artery are the two posterior cerebral arteries; one serves each side of the brain. A stroke involving these branches is likely to affect vision since the part of the cerebral hemisphere that processes vision is located in this part of the brain. This artery also serves the cerebellum, so disturbance of coordination or gait is also likely from a stroke in this blood vessel.

Perhaps more importantly, the basilar artery gives off small branches to all parts of the brain stem, providing the only blood supply to these areas. Strokes involving these blood vessels can cause widespread and bizarre combinations of symptoms, since so many fiber tracts travel through the brain stem on their way to the body. The brain stem also contains the centers of the brain that control breathing, blood pressure, and even consciousness. Thus strokes in this area are more likely to cause major medical problems and loss of consciousness than strokes originating in the carotid arteries.

EMBOLI AND MICROEMBOLI

An embolus (emboli is the plural of embolus) is any object that blocks blood flow through an artery. The most common type of emboli are blood clots, but emboli can also be bits of plaque or other types of tissue. The emboli that cause stroke most often arise from plaque in diseased arteries; they can also come from the heart or other parts of the body.

Any emboli that originate in the left side of the heart (the side that pumps blood from the lungs into the body) will pass directly into the aorta and then other arteries of the body. Because the brain receives a large portion of the body's blood flow, it is likely that at least some of these emboli will reach the small arteries of the brain and cause a stroke. People who have enlarged hearts, artificial heart valves, or atrial fibrillation (abnormal heart rhythm) are at high risk of forming such emboli.

Emboli originating in the legs or distant parts of the body are usually screened out by the lungs since blood returning to the heart from most parts of the body passes through the small capillaries of the lungs, where the emboli will lodge. For this reason blood clots originating in the veins of the legs can cause pulmonary emboli (emboli travelling to the lungs) but rarely stroke.

About 10 percent of people have a condition known as patent foramen ovale. In this condition an opening exists between the heart's left and right atria. This condition usually causes absolutely no symptoms, but it can allow an emboli to pass from the body into the left side of the heart without being screened out by the lungs. In this case, blood clots forming in the legs or other parts of the body could actually cause a stroke.

Microemboli are tiny bits of plaque that obstruct the smallest arteries of the brain. They can originate from disease in any of the brain's arteries, or from blood clots in the heart. Because the area of brain involved when a small artery is obstructed by a microembolus is quite small, people may not even realize they've had a stroke; other areas of the brain simply take over the function of the damaged area. The person suffering microemboli may realize something is wrong. They can develop problems with memory, don't think properly, or may have a bit of weakness or numbness in one part of the body. The symptoms usually go away in a few days, however, and the person may never seek medical attention for them.

If microemboli continue to form, the brain will slowly be destroyed, one small piece at a time. It is extremely important, therefore, that anyone having even vague neurologic symptoms get evaluated for possible cerebral vascular disease. Once the source of microemboli is found, further emboli can usually be prevented.

CEREBRAL HEMORRHAGE AND ANEURYSMS

Only 20 percent of strokes are caused by cerebral hemorrhage. Hemorrhagic strokes are generally classified into two types depending upon the actual location where bleeding occurred. Subarachnoid hemorrhage means the bleeding is outside the brain tissue, but within the dura (the membranes surrounding the brain). Subarachnoid hemorrhage is usually caused by a congenital (born with) abnormality in the blood vessels. In the vast majority of cases the abnormality is an aneurysm, a balloonlike weakening of the artery's wall. In a few cases, the abnormality is an arteriovenous malformation, an abnormal tangled group of blood vessels containing both arteries and veins. The walls of these blood vessels are very thin, like an aneurysm, and therefore likely to rupture.

Subarachnoid hemorrhage causes problems because the bleeding will fill the skull with blood and eventually compress brain tissue.

If this continues, the brain tissue can become so distorted that it tears. Additionally, if enough pressure builds up within the skull, it can prevent blood from entering the skull, thus cutting off circulation to the brain.

The second type of hemorrhage is an intracerebral hemorrhage, meaning the bleeding is occurring within the brain itself. This type of bleeding is most often caused by untreated high blood pressure, but can sometimes be caused by an aneurysm or arteriovenous malformation inside the brain tissue. When an intracerebral hemorrhage occurs, the bleeding stretches and tears brain tissue, causing some degree of permanent destruction. If the bleeding continues long enough, it can also cause problems identical to a subarachnoid hemorrhage.

Cerebral Infarction (Death of Brain Cells)

Whenever blood circulation to an area of the brain ceases, a series of events occur to the brain cells in that location. When circulation first ceases, the neurons (brain cells) in the affected area stop working to conserve the remaining oxygen. If oxygen is not restored, the neurons will begin to die within five to ten minutes. Once a neuron dies, it will never be replaced. Humans (like most animals) do not make new neurons after birth. In certain conditions, however, neurons in other areas of the brain can partially take over the functions of the destroyed neurons.

In most cases of ischemic stroke, the central area served by the blocked artery receives no blood flow at all, and neurons in this area all die within a few minutes. Brain tissue around this central area may receive some blood flow—enough to keep neurons alive—but not enough to allow them to function properly. If circulation to this area improves, these neurons can return to normal function and the amount of damage caused by the stroke is minimal. If circulation worsens, these neurons will also die and consequently the stroke will worsen.

Most of the immediate treatment following an ischemic stroke focuses on saving this area of marginal circulation around the center of the stroke. Just like any other tissue, brain tissue tends to swell when it becomes damaged. If substantial swelling occurs in the "marginal" area, the blood vessels will become even more obstructed and more neurons will die. If swelling can be prevented, then these neurons will have a much better chance of surviving.

Similarly, if circulation can be improved the neurons are more likely to return to normal function. Although it is usually not possible to surgically remove the clot responsible for a stroke, it may be possible to inject medications that can help it to dissolve. Doctors must do this soon after the stroke has occurred, however. If they wait too long, the blood vessels in the affected area can become so weak that they will rupture if circulation is restored, causing a cerebral hemorrhage.

The treatment of a hemorrhagic stroke is quite different. When a hemorrhagic stroke occurs, obviously the most important part of treatment is to stop the bleeding. This may be done by giving medication to lower blood pressure, but in some cases it requires emergency surgery. Even when the bleeding is stopped, however, other problems can occur. As the blood clot begins to dissolve, it will swell, causing more pressure on the brain. The blood clot can also irritate other arteries in the brain causing them to go into spasm. This spasm can be so severe that it causes an ischemic stroke in addition to the hemorrhagic stroke.

The Symptoms and Warning Signs of Stroke

The only symptom present in every type of stroke is some change in brain function. In large strokes or those involving the brain stem, the change may be a total loss of consciousness. In some very minor strokes caused by microemboli, the change may be only increased irritability, confusion, or a headache.

The symptoms of the stroke, and any warning signs that occur before it happens, vary depending upon the type of vascular problem that is present. In an embolic stroke there are usually no warning signs, although the person may know they have conditions that place them at risk or may have suffered a stroke in the past. In many strokes, however, the affected person had warning signs that were present for months before the actual stroke occurred.

SYMPTOMS OF EMBOLIC STROKES

The symptoms of embolic stroke usually develop suddenly over a few minutes, and then do not change for at least the first few hours after the stroke occurs. Embolic strokes rarely cause headache or any other pain. There are rarely any warning signs, but the person may have been advised they had heart disease or some other condition that could cause stroke. Exactly which symptoms an individual person develops once the stroke occurs varies depending upon which artery becomes obstructed.

If the stroke involves the internal carotid artery or the middle cerebral artery, the person becomes weak or numb on one side. If only one branch of the artery is involved, symptoms may be quite limited. It is common to develop weakness in just the arm, for example, or be unable to speak even though there is no paralysis. The stroke may also cause other abnormalities. The victim may have an area of vision (to one side, for example) that develops a blind spot, become unable to speak, or become unable to understand spoken words.

If the stroke involves the vertebral or basilar arteries, the symptoms may involve one or both sides of the body, or may not involve the body below the neck at all. Dizziness, difficulty walking or balancing, and numbness or weakness of the face are likely with these types of strokes. Unconsciousness and inability to focus the eyes (because the muscle controlling the eyes is weakened) are also common.

Strokes in these areas may also cause difficulty speaking but usually do not cause difficulty understanding spoken words.

SYMPTOMS OF ISCHEMIC STROKES

Ischemic strokes cause symptoms similar to embolic strokes, although they are more likely to involve large areas of the brain. An ischemic stroke may not begin as suddenly as an embolic stroke, however. Often they slowly become more severe over time, encompassing larger areas of the body, or over a few hours as new symptoms develop. Up to 40 percent of ischemic strokes gradually worsen for up to forty-eight hours.

More importantly, ischemic strokes are much more likely to give warning signs before the actual stroke occurs. The most important warning sign is called a Transient Ischemic Attack (commonly referred to as a TIA). A TIA is a short period during which part of the brain doesn't get enough oxygen.

A TIA can have all the initial symptoms of a stroke—weakness, numbness, difficulty speaking, even unconsciousness. Unlike a complete stroke, however, the symptoms of a TIA go away completely after a period of time, usually fifteen to thirty minutes but sometimes several hours. Many people who have a TIA decide not to get medical attention because their symptoms disappear completely after the event is over. In most cases, a person suffering a TIA will go on to develop a complete stroke within weeks or months if they do not get medical treatment.

In some cases, TIAs steadily become more frequent and longer lasting until finally a complete stroke develops. More commonly, a person has one or more TIAs and then suddenly develops a complete stroke. In still other cases, the person never suffers a TIA; their first symptom is a complete stroke.

CASE STUDY: Ischemic Stroke

Mark, a sixty-four-year-old retiree, had a heart attack and coronary artery bypass graft performed five years ago. He stopped smoking, began exercising, and has done well since that time. About three months ago, he noticed a tingling in his entire right arm and had trouble speaking for about fifteen minutes. Since the symptoms went away quickly, he assumed he'd had a bit too much of the Florida sunshine and didn't think about it again. The same symptoms returned about a month later but again stopped after fifteen minutes. A week after that they occurred for a third time, and Mark called his doctor and made an appointment for the following week.

Unfortunately, the next morning Mark could not move his right arm or leg, the left side of his face sagged weakly, and his speech was garbled. His wife called an ambulance and he was taken to the hospital. Doctors performed an MRI scan that was read as normal by the radiologist, but because of his clinical symptoms the doctors were certain he was having a stroke. Because the doctors could not be sure how long it had been since the stroke began, they could not risk using a "clot-busting" drug.

Mark was admitted to the stroke care unit of the hospital, and a repeat MRI scan the next morning confirmed he had a large stroke involving the left cerebral hemisphere. During that day his condition deteriorated and doctors place him on a ventilator and began medications to reduce swelling in his brain. Three days later, they were able let Mark breathe on his own again, and after two more days Mark was transferred to a regular hospital room. An arteriogram indicated that Mark had widespread cerebrovascular disease. Since his carotid arteries were not severely obstructed, doctors began treatment with aspirin to help prevent a future stroke.

Mark was then transferred to a rehabilitation hospital to begin recovery from his stroke. After six weeks, Mark could walk well, although he must wear a brace to support his right ankle. He still has some difficulty speaking—while his wife understands him perfectly, she must sometimes interpret his words for other people. Unfortunately, Mark's right arm is densely paralyzed, and doctors don't expect him to regain much use of his arm. He has been able to learn to shave and brush his teeth just fine with his left hand and is making some progress in learning to write with that hand.

SYMPTOMS OF A HEMORRHAGIC STROKE

The symptoms of a hemorrhagic stroke vary depending upon the cause of the hemorrhage and its location. When the stroke is caused by an aneurysm or arteriovenous malformation, the person may experience some warning signs before the hemorrhage occurs. If the aneurysm itself pushes on some structure in the brain, it may cause changes in vision, or weakness and numbness in an area of the body. When symptoms such as these do occur, they generally worsen over time until the aneurysm ruptures suddenly.

Actual rupture of the aneurysm causing a subarachnoid hemorrhage usually causes a sudden, extremely severe headache, though this doesn't always happen. There may not be any specific loss of function in a single area of the body (at least at first), but loss of consciousness, or at least altered consciousness, is common. Often, a person having a hemorrhagic stroke will become nauseous or vomit. Unlike embolic and ischemic strokes, the symptoms of strokes caused by subarachnoid hemorrhage slowly and steadily worsen over time. For example, a person suffering a hemorrhagic stroke might suddenly develop a horrible headache and become nauseous. Within an hour or less they might begin feeling very sleepy or not thinking clearly. Soon after, the person might have total loss of consciousness or begin to have signs of paralysis.

Persons with intracerebral hemorrhage caused by hypertension are less likely to have warning signs, although many will know that they have high blood pressure. (It is possible to have an intracerebral hemorrhage with normal blood pressure, however). A headache often occurs with intracerebral hemorrhage but may not be more severe than a routine tension headache.

Unlike subarachnoid hemorrhage, an intracerebral hemorrhage usually causes a sudden neurologic problem, such as paralysis, dizziness, inability to focus the eyes, weakness, numbness, or sometimes even pain in one part of the body. Drowsiness is common, as is nausea and vomiting. Complete loss of consciousness usually doesn't occur, however. In some cases, the person will have a seizure.

The symptoms will generally worsen over time, but not nearly as fast as the symptoms of subarachnoid hemorrhage. In fact, it isn't uncommon for persons with intracerebral hemorrhage to have slowly worsening symptoms lasting more than a day before they decide to go to the hospital.

CASE STUDY: Hemorrhagic Stroke

James, a forty-nine-year-old, has been nagged by his doctor and his wife for years to lose weight and get some exercise. He's had high blood pressure for several years, but isn't very good about taking his medicine, since he really doesn't feel any better after taking it. Two months ago his health insurance changed. It no longer paid for his blood pressure medicine. Since the medication was quite expensive, James decided to just stop taking it.

For two days James had a pretty bad headache and felt sick to his stomach. Yesterday he threw up twice in the morning and stayed home from work. He noticed he had trouble reading since the print seemed a little blurry, so he just watched television and napped. Last night, his headache suddenly got much worse. He also became confused and very sleepy. His wife called an ambulance and James was taken to the hospital.

In the emergency room, James's blood pressure was found to be extremely high. He was given medication to lower his blood pressure and an emergency CT scan was performed. The scan revealed that James had an intracerebral hemorrhage (bleeding within the brain). James's blood pressure has been under good control overnight, but he remains confused. A repeat CT scan this morning showed the bleeding hasn't worsened, however, and doctors expect a full recovery.

OTHER CONDITIONS THAT MIMIC STROKE

There are a few other conditions that cause symptoms similar to stroke. However, it is important to remember that if you think you may be having a stroke, you should go immediately to the nearest hospital. Waiting to see if the symptoms will go away is the likeliest way to insure that you suffer a severe stroke, perhaps one that could have been entirely prevented.

In any case, most of the conditions that appear similar to a stroke are also medical emergencies that require treatment. For example, infection of the brain (encephalitis) or the lining of the brain (meningitis) can cause symptoms similar to a stroke. In most cases, however, infection also causes fever and chills, as well as other symptoms associated with infection.

Only very rarely will a migraine headache cause changes in vision, weakness, or paralysis that is very similar to a stroke. A person having a seizure may lose consciousness briefly and have partial paralysis once they regain consciousness. If the seizure was not witnessed by anyone, it may appear very similar to a stroke. Diabetics who take too much insulin will have strokelike symptoms because their blood sugar level is too low for the brain to function normally. Finally, brain tumors may cause bleeding that is exactly the same as an intracerebral hemorrhage.

All these are very serious medical conditions that require immediate medical attention. There are no conditions similar to a stroke that should be "watched" to see if they go away.

CHAPTER 6

Treatment and Prevention of Cerebrovascular Disease and Stroke

Stroke Risk Factors

Anyone can have a stroke, but the presence of several different factors, some of which are unavoidable, but many of which can be changed or modified (see Table 6.1 on page 83), make a person much more likely to have a stroke. In fact, an individual's risk of having a stroke can be predicted quite accurately simply by knowing which risk factors are present. For example, a seventy-year-old male smoker with high blood pressure who has had a heart attack in the past has a 14 percent chance of having a stroke during the next ten years; a seventy-two-year-old female with diabetes has a 9 percent chance of having a stroke during the same time period.

Obviously, some risk factors, such as a person's age or a family history of stroke, cannot be changed. Others, such as chronic exposure to cold, are easily changed, while still others, such as high blood pressure and cigarette smoking, can be changed with some difficulty. It is important to realize that risk factors compound each other. For example, if you have a family history of stroke, smoking raises your risk far more than it would for a person with no family history of stroke.

The three major risk factors that can be minimized for persons at risk of having a stroke are high blood pressure, smoking, and atherosclerosis. Atherosclerosis, commonly called "hardening of the arteries," is described in detail in chapter 5. We know that atherosclerosis is much more likely to develop in people who smoke, have high levels of cholesterol and fat in their blood, don't exercise, and have a family history of the disease. Except for family history, these factors can all be reduced by lifestyle changes and medications.

Any risk factor that is treated will significantly lower a person's risk of having a stroke. Such treatment can range from delicate surgery to remove plaques from blood vessels to medications that lower blood pressure or cholesterol. More important than any of these, however, are the simple lifestyle changes that anyone can make—quitting smoking, losing weight, and exercising.

In addition to general lifestyle changes and medical treatment for atherosclerosis, prevention of stroke in most people will also involve some medical treatment to minimize the likelihood that blood clots will form over the diseased arteries. For people who are at risk of embolic stroke—a stroke resulting from a piece of blood clot breaking off and blocking a distant artery in the brain—medical treatment may be the most important method of preventing strokes.

People who have significant atherosclerosis in the carotid artery may require surgery to remove the plaque and widen the artery. Although such surgery (discussed below) is not without its risks, in many cases the risk of carotid artery surgery is far lower than that of stroke if the plaque is not treated. When disease involves the vertebral or basilar arteries, surgery is usually impossible because of the location of these blood vessels. In these cases, medical treatment is usually the only therapy possible.

Persons at risk of either ischemic or embolic stroke will usually require several of the treatments discussed in this chapter. For this rea-

Table 6.1   Risk Factors Associated with Suffering a Stroke

High Risk	Moderate Risk
High blood pressure	Oral contraceptive use
Heart disease of any type	Migraine headaches with aura
Cigarette smoking	High blood cholesterol or
Carotid artery vascular disease	triglycerides
History of transient ischemic attack	Chronic exposure to cold
Age greater than 60 (risk increases as age advances)	Black race
Family history of stroke	

son, all the various treatments used to prevent stroke in people at risk of ischemic stroke are discussed together. The exact treatments used, however, will vary depending upon the location and severity of the vascular disease, as well as other medical problems the patient may have.

People at risk of hemorrhage from an aneurysm or arteriovenous malformation will usually require surgery to correct the problem. Aneurysm surgery is more complex and has a higher risk of complications than does carotid artery surgery—especially if the aneurysm has already ruptured. Persons with aneurysm or arteriovenous malformations usually do not have atherosclerosis or other cerebrovascular disease, however. Since the treatment of these problems is quite different than the treatment of cerebrovascular disease, it is discussed separately at the end of this chapter.

Effects of Lifestyle Changes

Lifestyle changes can dramatically affect two of the major risk factors for stroke: atherosclerosis and high blood pressure. Although these changes are rather simple to write about, they are hard to put into

practice. If a person is motivated, though, they can dramatically reduce their risk of stroke. Many studies have shown that making simple lifestyle changes, such as those described here, can cut a person's
stroke risk in half in a period of a few months.

EXERCISE AND DIET

Diet

The amount of total cholesterol, saturated fat, and total fat that you
eat all affect your blood cholesterol and triglyceride levels. Changing
your diet can dramatically reduce the levels of both substances in your
blood, thus reducing one of the primary risk factors for developing
atherosclerosis.

Most dietary changes focus on lowering the amount of cholesterol
and saturated fat consumed. In the body, cholesterol exists in two
forms: Low Density Lipoprotein (LDL) and High Density Lipoprotein (HDL). LDL is commonly called "bad" cholesterol because it
carries cholesterol to atherosclerotic plaques in the arteries (as well as
other locations). HDL is "good" cholesterol because it carries cholesterol to the liver where it is broken down and destroyed.

The typical American diet contains huge amounts of fat—about
38 percent of all calories consumed are in the form of fats. We also eat
large amounts of cholesterol, about 440 mg per day on average, which
is far more than people in most other countries consume.

All our cholesterol intake comes from animal products. Red meat,
poultry, and most fish contain significant amounts of cholesterol, as
does whole milk. The meats derived from animal organs—brains,
liver, kidneys, and sweetbreads—are extremely high in cholesterol.
Egg yolks contain probably the highest amount of cholesterol of any
food, between 210 and 250 mg in each yolk. Since most diets recommend less than 300 mg of cholesterol a day, egg yolks must be almost
totally eliminated if you want a healthy diet. Egg whites, however, are
low in cholesterol, as are egg substitute products.

Saturated fat also raises the level of LDL cholesterol, and reducing the amount of saturated fat is another major goal of a healthy diet. In general, beef, pork, poultry, milk, and eggs all contain significant amounts of saturated fat. Some vegetable oils contain very little saturated fat, while other types of vegetable oil contain huge amounts of saturated fat. Coconut and palm oil, for example, contain more saturated fat than butter or lard. Corn and safflower oils, on the other hand, contain mostly unsaturated fat.

Dietary recommendations for each person can vary widely depending upon body size, exercise level, and the presence of certain diseases. In general, however, anyone at significant risk of stroke (and anyone who has already suffered a stroke) should make as many positive changes in their diet as they can (see appendix A).

It is important to remember that all fried foods contain large amounts of oil, no matter how carefully they are dried after frying. Potatoes, for example, contain almost no fat, but an order of french fries may contain thirty or more grams of fat—half an entire day's allotment for most reasonable diets. This is especially important to remember when eating fried restaurant food since commercial oils used by restaurants are usually made from palm oil, coconut oil, and animal fats, all of which contain large amounts of saturated fat.

Specific dietary recommendations for each person will vary, but anyone with vascular disease should make as many positive changes in their diet as they can. Specifically, a diet for a person at risk of stroke should be similar to that described in the "moderate cholesterol reduction" diet, while persons with undesirable lipid profiles should consider a "strict cholesterol reduction" diet (see Table 6.2). Simply reading labels and avoiding the worst offending ingredients listed on page 87 will dramatically improve the diet of most people.

Generally, a healthy diet will begin to lower blood cholesterol level within two to three weeks. Most Americans can easily obtain approximately a 10 percent reduction in serum cholesterol from their diet alone. Since the risk of future vascular disease can be reduced

Table 6.2   Moderate and Strict Cholesterol Reduction Diets

	Moderate	Strict
Total Fat (% of calories)	30%	<30%
Saturated	<10%	<7%
Polyunsaturated	10%	10%
Monounsaturated	10–15%	10–15%
Cholesterol Intake	<300 mg/day	<200 mg/day

Note: Total calories will vary depending on body size, activity level, and need to lose weight.

twice as much as the percent reduction in cholesterol, dietary changes alone can result in a 20 percent reduction in stroke risk.

Eating foods that contain water soluble fiber (such as oat bran) will also lower the blood cholesterol level. One study determined that men eating 100 g of water soluble fiber a day had a decrease in cholesterol levels of almost 20 percent. This fiber can be taken as a dietary supplement, since a wide variety of powdered fiber products are available. It can also be obtained by eating fiber-rich brans, fruits, and vegetables.

Lack of Exercise

A sedentary lifestyle—one with very little exercise—predisposes people to atherosclerosis and worsens high blood pressure. The Framingham Heart Study, a study that followed several thousand people for many years to determine the various factors that constituted risks for heart disease, found that inactive people are five times more likely to have a heart attack, and more than twice as likely to have a stroke, than are those who exercise regularly.

Not exercising increases levels of LDL ("bad" cholesterol) in the bloodstream and lowers levels of HDL ("good" cholesterol). When people who have inactive lifestyles begin to exercise regularly, they lower their total cholesterol and increase their HDL cholesterol. Exercise is especially beneficial for postmenopausal women. Women who exercise regularly after menopause have much lower total cholesterol and higher HDL levels than women who don't exercise.

People who don't exercise are also more likely to develop high blood pressure than those who do. Even if a person already has high blood pressure, they can still benefit from exercise. Studies have shown that people with mild to moderate hypertension (diastolic blood pressure of 90 to 100) require less medication once they have started an exercise program.

The most important type of exercise for people at risk of stroke (and heart disease for that matter) is aerobic exercise—basically any form of exercise that raises your pulse rate and makes you breathe faster. Walking, swimming, even

> ### KEY INGREDIENTS TO AVOID
>
> - Any animal fat (including chicken fat)
> - Chocolate or cocoa butter
> - Coconut or coconut oil
> - Egg or egg solids
> - Hydrogenated fat or oil
> - Lard
> - Lauric acid
> - Mysteric acid
> - Palm or palm kernel oil
> - Palmitic acid
> - Shortening
> - Vegetable fat*
> - Vegetable shortening*
> - Whole milk solids
>
> *When this label is used, the product usually has palm or coconut oil. If the manufacturer used the more expensive "healthy" vegetable oils, they would almost certainly advertise it.

wading back and forth in the shallow end of a swimming pool are excellent forms of aerobic exercise. Golf (at least when using a cart) and weight lifting are not. As little as fifteen minutes of aerobic exercise three times a week (a good starting point for most people) will have a beneficial effect. Most physicians suggest an end point of thirty to sixty minutes of aerobic activity four times a week, although some recommend daily exercise.

It takes some time for many people to accustom themselves to exercise this much. Most medical literature suggests a period of six to eight weeks for inactive people to raise their level of exercise. Persons who have diabetes, heart trouble, or severe arthritis should consult with their doctor about what type of exercise is most appropriate for them.

The benefits of exercise increase over time. Many studies show that cholesterol levels and blood pressure drop steadily during the first year of an exercise program. If a person stops exercising, however, the benefits will reverse themselves. After six to eight weeks without exercise, most people will begin to show a slow increase in cholesterol, blood pressure, and weight.

SMOKING

The Risk of Smoking

Smoking is a very high-risk habit, not only increasing the chance of stroke but also heart disease, several types of cancer, and emphysema. According to the Surgeon General, 20 percent of all deaths in the U.S. are the result of diseases caused by cigarette smoking. Smoking directly causes about a half million deaths per year in the U.S., more than AIDS, drug abuse (including alcohol abuse and drunk driving), and all accidents combined.

In general, smokers are at least twice as likely to develop coronary artery disease and almost twice as likely to have a stroke. The risk is also proportional to the number of years smoked: someone who has smoked for twenty years has twice the risk of someone who has smoked for ten years.

No one is absolutely certain what substances in cigarette smoke are the most harmful, since tobacco smoke contains over 4,000 different chemicals that are absorbed by the body. We do know that something in tobacco smoke increases the risk of atherosclerosis (hardening of the arteries). Smoking also increases the blood's tendency to form clots over plaques, raising the risk of heart attack and stroke once atherosclerosis has occurred. There is some evidence that a chemical in tobacco smoke also damages the lining of blood vessels, making clots even more likely to occur.

Additionally, nicotine increases blood pressure, adding further to the risk of stroke. Smoke also contains carbon monoxide, which reduces the blood's ability to carry oxygen, meaning that even less oxygen can be delivered to the brain. Nicotine and carbon monoxide also cause the arteries to constrict. If a diseased artery constricts, its diameter may narrow until it can't deliver blood to the brain, causing a TIA or even a stroke.

Smoking not only has direct effects that increase the risk of stroke, it is associated with raising other risk factors such as the development of heart disease and rising cholesterol levels as well. Smoking is especially dangerous for people who already have other risk factors such as diabetes or a strong family history of stroke. Smoking increases the risk of stroke by about 40 percent for men and 60 percent for women. (The risk of stroke increases in women because smoking offsets the beneficial effects of estrogen, in addition to causing the same changes that it does in men.)

About Quitting Cigarettes

People who stop smoking can lower their risk of stroke dramatically. In fact, beneficial changes can be detected within a few days of quitting. For example, carbon monoxide levels in the blood begin to drop within two days of quitting and within thirty days are almost undetectable. Blood pressure usually drops slightly within seven days of quitting. Oxygen levels in the blood increase within four to five days of quitting.

Many smokers are surprised to find that they actually cough a bit more right after they quit. This is because cigarette smoke actually suppresses the cough reflex. (Not having a cigarette all night is one reason for the morning "smoker's cough" some people have.) The cough goes away in two to three months. Improvement in lung function continues for the next six months, and the level of cholesterol in the blood drops during the same time. Two years after quitting, an ex-smoker is only slightly more at risk of having a stroke than people who have never smoked. After five years, the risk of stroke is no higher than for people who have never smoked.

As all smokers know, quitting is easier said than done. Nicotine is a drug that affects many organs in the body, including the brain. Over time the brain develops a physical dependence on nicotine; it becomes used to the drug's presence and brain function is altered for a while when the drug is removed. Withdrawal symptoms usually begin within a few hours after quitting smoking and don't reach their peak for several days.

The most noticeable symptom of nicotine withdrawal is a craving for cigarettes. Other common symptoms include restlessness, difficulty sleeping, anxiety, irritability, headache, difficulty concentrating, and sometimes mild depression. The major symptoms last from one week to two weeks, but they may return as periods of "secondary withdrawal" for several months. Secondary withdrawal symptoms usually last only a few hours, or a day at most.

The good news is that there are a lot of things that can be done to help someone quit smoking. In fact, there are books and seminars devoted to just that topic. There is no way to cover all that material here, and it is strongly suggested that you investigate these other sources for further help.

It is important to enlist the help and support of people around you when attempting to quit. The key words are "support" and "attempt." It is important for family and friends to be understanding while you are trying to stop, and it is also important that they realize nagging a person who is undergoing nicotine withdrawal is not very helpful.

Quitting "cold turkey," that is, giving up cigarettes and tolerating the withdrawal symptoms until they pass, is successful for a lot of people. Many others find that they are unable to tolerate the withdrawal symptoms without other forms of help, however. Nicotine replacement therapy, medications to ease withdrawal symptoms, support groups, hypnosis, and a variety of "stop smoking" programs have all had success. There is no single easy way to quit. Overall, none of these techniques is much more successful than any other. Whatever method you use to quit, remember that the average smoker makes between three and four attempts to quit before they are finally successful.

Nicotine replacement therapy is available in the form of nicotine gum or nicotine skin patches. Replacement therapy provides a dose of nicotine similar to what you would get from smoking, and thus eliminates the physical withdrawal symptoms during the period of breaking the smoking habit.

Each form of therapy has its advantages. The gum can be used as needed, mimicking the intermittent doses of nicotine that a person would get from smoking cigarettes. The major disadvantage of gum is that the dose is not very well regulated. Chewing the gum vigorously can deliver very high levels of nicotine. Some people also find that the gum irritates the inside of their mouth and are unable to use it for this reason.

Nicotine patches have the advantage of delivering an accurate, constant level of nicotine to the bloodstream. They also are available in various strengths, allowing a well-regulated tapering of the nicotine dose. Some smokers find that the steady level of nicotine delivered by patches does not stop their withdrawal as well as the variable levels supplied by nicotine gum, however.

There are also many types of smoking cessation groups. Some are run by insurance companies or hospitals and are free or available at very low cost. Others are for-profit groups that charge a significant fee. The success rates of these groups are usually higher than those experienced by smokers trying to quit by themselves. None of them have long-term success rates of even 50 percent, however, and no reputable program will make such a claim. Any group that charges a large fee and promises spectacular success rates should be viewed with suspicion.

Other people swear by the success of hypnosis, acupuncture, special diets, and herbal remedies. Scientifically, none of these techniques has been rigorously tested, and some of the claims made for them appear ridiculously inflated. Nevertheless, any therapy that helps you to quit is a great therapy, and certainly none of them do anything that would be considered harmful.

Treatment for Medical Conditions

While lifestyle changes can effectively reduce the risk of stroke, some people have serious medical conditions that also increase their risk of stroke. Others will require medical therapy to treat atherosclerosis that has already developed, or that is too severe to treat by diet and exercise alone. Since a person who has recovered from a stroke is at high risk of another stroke, they will usually be given medication to help reduce this risk.

MEDICATIONS

The medical therapy used to reduce the risk of stroke is directed to achieve one of three major goals: halting the progression of atherosclerosis, preventing blood clots from developing, and controlling high blood pressure. Since many people have several conditions that place them at risk for stroke, it isn't uncommon for them to take several different medications. For the most part, these medicines must be taken daily for the rest of the person's life.

MEDICATIONS USED TO
PREVENT ATHEROSCLEROSIS

Whenever atherosclerosis has been found in one part of the body, it probably also exists in many other parts. A person who has had a heart attack from coronary artery disease (atherosclerosis in the arteries going to the heart) probably also has some cerebral vascular disease (atherosclerosis in the arteries going to the brain).

Medical treatment does not really affect the atherosclerotic plaques directly. Rather it is aimed at reducing bad cholesterol (LDL) and fats in the bloodstream, while increasing levels of good cholesterol (HDL). It has been shown that if these changes are made, the atherosclerotic plaques will stop growing. In some cases the plaques actually shrink and the arteries return to almost normal condition.

Treating atherosclerosis with medication is not required in all cases. Many people are able to make these changes by implementing a proper diet, exercising, and quitting cigarettes. Others, especially those with a strong family history, will require medications to reduce their LDL and fat levels to an acceptable range.

Medications are used when dietary changes and exercise do not sufficiently reduce triglycerides and cholesterol in the blood to safe levels. For people with severe elevations of cholesterol or triglycerides, medications may be used immediately in addition to dietary changes. They are also indicated in people who have hereditary conditions that cause elevated cholesterol or triglyceride levels.

A variety of drugs can be used to lower the levels of cholesterol and fats in the bloodstream. Each has different effects and side effects, and most people will have to try a couple of these medications before they find one that is both effective and well tolerated.

Bile Acid Sequestrants   Bile acid sequestrants include cholestyramine (Questran®, Cholybar®) and colestipol (Colestid®). These medications trap the bile (one of the digestive chemicals) in the intestines and prevent the body from reabsorbing it. Since bile contains a lot of cholesterol, these medications will actually remove cholesterol from the body. Most people experience gas, abdominal cramps, and constipation when they start taking these drugs, but the symptoms usually stop after a few weeks.

Bile acid sequestrants are very likely to bind to other medications taken by mouth, thus preventing their absorption. For this reason, many doctors try not to use this class of cholesterol-reducing drugs in people who take several other medications. When they are used, however, bile acid sequestrants usually result in a drop of serum cholesterol of 10 to 20 percent. They do not affect the levels of triglycerides, nor do they change the proportions of HDL and LDL cholesterol.

Enzyme Blocking Agents   The most commonly used enzyme blockers include lovastatin (Mevacor®), pravastatin (Pravachol®), and simvastatin (Zocor®). These drugs interfere with an enzyme that manufactures cholesterol in the body. They selectively lower the levels of LDL (bad) cholesterol and triglycerides (fats) without lowering the level of HDL. Because they selectively reduce LDL, many doctors prefer them to other types of cholesterol reducing drugs.

These medications are likely to cause mild muscle pain, weakness, and headache at first, but these symptoms usually clear up in a week or two. In a few people they may cause blurred vision, headaches, stomach upset, and interfere with liver function. They can also interfere with medications, such as warfarin, that prevent the blood from clotting.

Niacin (Nia-Bid®, Nicobid®, Nicolar®, and others) is a medication that inhibits different enzymes. The major effect of this drug is to lower triglycerides, but it also lowers LDL cholesterol and may raise HDL (good) cholesterol. Though niacin causes few side effects, most people report feeling warm and flushed for a short time after taking it. You can take one aspirin to prevent this reaction thirty minutes before taking the niacin. In a very few cases, niacin interferes with liver function, so your doctor may order blood tests a month or two after you've begun the medication.

Other Medications   Clofibrate (Atromid-S®) is a medication used to lower triglycerides in the blood, although no one understands exactly how it works. To a lesser extent, clofibrate also lowers cholesterol levels. Clofibrate is most commonly used for people who have genetically high triglyceride levels. Many people have muscle pain and weakness when they first take clofibrate, but this usually clears up in a few weeks. People taking the drug must have periodic blood tests for liver function since it can interfere with the liver.

Gemfibrozil (Lopid®) also lowers triglycerides by an unknown mechanism. The possible side effects of gemfibrozil are similar to those of the enzyme-blocking drugs: muscle pain, blurred vision, insomnia, headaches, and stomach upset.

Medications Used to Prevent Thrombosis and Embolism

When an atherosclerotic plaque becomes large enough, it destroys the normal smooth lining of the artery, leaving a roughened surface. The blood exposed to this surface will eventually form a clot (called a thrombus) over the plaque. The thrombus may completely block the blood vessel causing a thrombotic stroke, or pieces of the clot may break off, blocking a smaller blood artery as a result and causing an embolic stroke.

To help prevent thrombosis and embolism, most people with cerebral vascular disease will take some medication to slow down the blood's clotting mechanisms. These medications are often referred to as "blood thinners," although they really don't thin the blood at all. They just make it less likely to clot.

Aspirin is by far the most widely prescribed medicine to prevent thrombosis. It works by interfering with small particles in the blood called platelets that are involved in the first steps of blood clotting. A single baby aspirin a day is sufficient to block platelets as much as possible. Taking more aspirin is fine if you get a headache, but it does not provide any additional anticlotting activity.

An alternative to aspirin is ticlopidine. Ticlopidine has a similar effect on platelets, and several studies suggest it is better than aspirin at preventing stroke. Unfortunately, the medication has severe side effects in a few (about 0.5 percent) people who take it, and it is quite expensive. For this reason, aspirin is still the most widely prescribed drug for inhibiting platelets.

In some cases stronger anticoagulants (medications that prevent blood from clotting) are indicated. This is usually required when a person suffers an embolic stroke arising from the heart or other part of the body. These medications do not interfere with platelets but instead prevent the chemicals in the blood that form the actual clot from working. Dosages of all these medications must be carefully individualized. Your doctor will prescribe a dose that should be effective, and after a week or so will measure the blood's actual clotting ability. Should there be too much or not enough anticlotting effect, the dosage will have to be adjusted.

Medications commonly used for this type of anticoagulation are warfarin, coumadin, and dicoumaral. All these drugs are quite similar and have similar side effects. By far the most significant side effect is abnormal bleeding. People taking these medicines bruise easily and bleed freely from even minor cuts. Although this is generally not dangerous, the medicine must be discontinued before even a minor surgical procedure.

Antihypertensive Medication

Hundreds of medications are used to treat high blood pressure, and discussing them individually would entail far too much time. The most important point to remember is that with so many medications to choose from, everyone should be able to find one that effectively lowers their blood pressure without causing side effects. Stopping a blood pressure medicine because of side effects is dangerous; chances are your blood pressure will become higher than it was before you began medication. Instead, simply notify your doctor of the problem you are having and ask him to try a different medication.

Other Medications

The other medications used to treat people at heightened risk of stroke are generally reserved for people who have an enlarged heart or abnormal heart rhythm that makes them likely to develop blood clots in the heart. These clots can give rise to large emboli that can cause massive strokes. Most people with these conditions will also take an oral anticoagulant to minimize the blood's ability to clot (see above).

People with atrial fibrillation, an abnormal heart rhythm in which the upper chambers of the heart (the atria) don't beat properly, may require medication to restore their heart to a normal rhythm. Quinidine (Cardioquin®, Duraquin®, Quinaglute®, Quinidex®, Quinalin®) is the most widely used of these medications. Procainamide (Procan SR®, Pronestyl®) is also used frequently, as is disopyramide (Norpace®, Norpace CR®).

Quindine can cause several side effects although most are not severe. Many people taking quinidine will experience intestinal cramps and diarrhea, and a few experience nausea and vomiting. These symptoms usually go away within three weeks after starting the medication. Procainamide can cause an allergic reaction including rash, chest or joint pain, and even blisters. Disopyramide can worsen congestive heart failure symptoms in patients with weakened heart muscles. It can also cause dry mouth and difficulty in urinating.

SURGERY FOR VASCULAR DISEASE

The only surgical procedure performed frequently to prevent strokes is carotid endarterectomy, the surgical removal of plaques from the carotid artery. Near the angle of the jaw, the carotid artery divides into two branches: the external carotid artery, which carries blood to the face and head, and the internal carotid artery, which carries blood to the brain. Atherosclerosis is most likely to develop at the area where the carotid divides. This area is easy to reach surgically, and the plaque can be removed from this location.

If the plaque becomes large enough to block 75 percent of the carotid artery, blood flow to the brain will be reduced. Any person with 75 percent narrowing of the carotid artery (usually called stenosis by doctors) should probably have surgery to correct the problem. Smaller plaques can be a problem if they become cracked and rough since this can cause thrombosis and emboli. People who have less than 75 percent stenosis but who have had a stroke or transient ischemic attacks (see chapter 5) may also be candidates for surgery.

Carotid Endarterectomy

Carotid endarterectomy is a fairly simple surgical procedure that involves removing the plaque from the inside of the carotid artery. It can be done under local anesthesia, but most people have general anesthesia for the operation.

The surgery itself is fairly straightforward. The surgeon makes an incision in the skin over the artery and then places clamps on the artery above and below the area where the plaque is located. Once the clamps are in place to prevent bleeding, the surgeon opens the artery and removes all the plaque. The artery is stitched back together, and the clamps are then removed, restoring circulation to the brain.

While the procedure is straightforward, it requires a high degree of skill to delicately remove the plaque without damaging the inside of the artery. It also requires speed on the part of the surgeon. During the time the artery is clamped, the carotid artery on that side is not delivering any blood flow to the brain. In theory, the other carotid artery and the basilar artery will deliver enough blood to prevent the brain from becoming damaged during the "clamp time," but obviously the surgeon will attempt to keep this period as short as possible.

Risks and Benefits of Surgery   There are several risks that accompany carotid endarterectomy. The period of cross clamping can cause a stroke to occur if the remaining circulation to the brain isn't sufficient. Should a piece of plaque become broken off by either the clamps or the surgery itself, the fragment can become an embolus and cause a stroke in one of the smaller arteries. Additionally, a strong anticoagulant is administered during surgery to prevent blood from clotting while the artery is clamped. This can cause bleeding in another part of the body.

Overall, however, the risk of complications during endarterectomy is about 3 percent, and most of those that do occur are not extremely severe. Patients being considered for endarterectomy have such a high risk of stroke that the risk of complications from endarterectomy are much lower than their risk of having a stroke if surgery is not performed.

Two large multicenter studies have been undertaken in recent years to decide when a person should have carotid endarterectomy: the North American Symptomatic Carotid Endarterectomy Trial (NASCET) and the European Carotid Surgery Trial (ECST). Both studies found that for people with 70 percent or greater obstruction of the carotid artery who also had a TIA or other stroke warning sign, the risk of stroke was reduced by two-thirds after carotid endarterectomy. For patients with similar obstruction but no warning signs, the risk was reduced by one-half.

Recovery After Surgery

Recovery from endarterectomy is usually quick and straightforward. During the first twenty-four hours the patient is often (but not always) monitored in an intensive care unit to insure no complications develop. Most people are discharged home within forty-eight to seventy-two hours and can resume normal activity within a few days. Most doctors do not want patients to drive for a few weeks after endarterectomy because of the risk that an accident could tear the stitches from surgery.

Most people who have had an endarterectomy will continue to take some medication to prevent blood clotting after surgery, but in most cases it will be only an aspirin a day. It is extremely important that patients with high blood pressure take their medication after endarterectomy surgery since high blood pressure could cause bleeding around the stitches in the carotid artery.

Angioplasty

An alternative to endarterectomy that can sometimes be used is called angioplasty. Angioplasty is not surgery in the true sense, but rather is a procedure done under x-ray guidance. It involves inserting a special catheter through an artery in the groin or arm and threading the catheter until it has reached the area of plaque in the carotid artery. A balloon at the end of the catheter is then blown up, flattening the plaque and opening the artery.

Although angioplasty does have a slightly lower complication rate than surgery, it is not risk-free. The catheter may break off bits of plaque, resulting in an embolus. It may even damage the lining of the artery, thus causing further obstruction. Bleeding can also occur in the artery where the catheter has been inserted. The major drawback to angioplasty is that it doesn't always work effectively, in which case the angioplasty will need to be repeated or an endarterectomy performed.

Treatment of Cerebral Aneurysm and Arteriovenous Malformations

In most cases, the first sign of an aneurysm or arteriovenous malformation is cerebral hemorrhage when the blood vessel has ruptured. Some other cases are discovered before rupture, either because they cause symptoms by pushing on the brain, or because they have been discovered almost by accident on a CT or MRI scan performed for some other reason. When an unruptured aneurysm is found, the treatment depends upon its size and location in the brain.

Arteriovenous malformations (AVM), which consist of a tangled mass of blood vessels, are more likely to cause symptoms before they actually rupture. Depending upon their size and location, they may be removed by surgery. The surgery involved begins with a craniotomy: removing a section of the skull to be able to operate directly on the brain. The surgeon must then find all the arteries going into the AVM and all the veins leaving it. The surgeon then clamps and ties each of these vessels before removing the malformation. Obviously, this surgery is prolonged and delicate. If the AVM is located deep within the brain, the surgery will also involve cutting through normal brain tissue to get to the area involved, making the procedure even more difficult.

If the AVM cannot be removed surgically, either because it is located deep in the brain or because the patient is too ill to withstand the surgery, a procedure much like angioplasty may be performed. A catheter is threaded from the large artery in the groin until it reaches an artery going into the AVM. A chemical that causes embolization is then injected through the catheter, causing the artery leading to the AVM to fill with clot, blocking blood flow into the AVM. In many cases, this will shrink the AVM enough to stop the symptoms and prevent the chance it will rupture. The procedure is not without risk, however, since the emboli may also cause a small stroke in areas of the brain near the AVM.

Another alternative is to use a special form of equipment, called a gamma knife, to focus a beam of radiation onto the AVM. Because blood vessels are very sensitive to this form of radiation, it can often destroy the AVM without harming brain tissue in the area. Gamma knife procedures only work on small AVMs, however.

Unlike AVMS, aneurysms do not always have to be removed. About 5 percent of otherwise normal people have small aneurysms in the blood vessels of the brain. Small aneurysms very rarely rupture, and usually the only treatment involved when a small aneurysm is discovered is to repeat an arteriogram or MRI scan in a few months to insure that the aneurysm is not growing. The larger the aneurysm the more likely it is to rupture, however, and once an aneurysm is more than 10 mm in diameter (about ¼ inch), surgery is usually indicated.

As with AVMs, surgery for an aneurysm requires a craniotomy. The aneurysm is not removed but rather a surgical clip is placed along its base, closing the aneurysm off from the artery. Even in the most experienced hands, aneurysm surgery has significant risks. The actual risk varies depending upon the location of the aneurysm, but about 3 percent of people overall will have some form of brain damage after aneurysm surgery. In most cases, this damage is minor and patients do recover. This risk is much less than that of death or major brain damage if a large aneurysm is left untreated, however.

Recently, attempts have been made to embolize aneurysms through arterial catheters. Various techniques have been recommended, including placing grafts inside the artery, using a "superglue" to fill up the aneurysm, and many others. The techniques involved in this procedure are still new, and at this time it is not clear which technique is best for which type of aneurysm. It is also not clear when these procedures should be used instead of surgery. Because of the risk involved in aneurysm surgery, however, the techniques are already being used frequently.

CHAPTER 7

The Diagnosis of Stroke

As discussed in chapter 5, the initial symptoms of a stroke vary greatly depending upon which area of the brain is involved, and the actual cause of the stroke. Because symptoms vary, it may be difficult to be absolutely certain that you are having a stroke. In severe cases, a stroke victim may suddenly and completely lose consciousness. When this occurs it can be difficult to determine if a stroke, massive heart attack, seizure, or some other problem is responsible. When the stroke involves only a small area of the brain, the symptoms may be so mild (a bit of slurred speech, or weakness in one eye for example) that the person may wait hours before seeking medical attention in hopes that the symptoms will pass.

If you have even the slightest suspicion that someone may be having a stroke, they should be taken immediately by ambulance to the nearest emergency room. Modern treatment can minimize a stroke's effects, and actually reverse the stroke in some cases, but treatment must be initiated very soon after the symptoms have started in order to be effective.

The Initial Symptoms of Stroke

When doctors first evaluate a person who has the symptoms of a stroke, they begin by assuming a stroke has occurred—but at the same time try to rule out any other possible cause. Diabetes with blood sugar that is too high or too low, a brain tumor, persons with epilepsy after a seizure, certain types of infection, and migraine attacks can all appear very similar to a stroke. In all these cases (except migraine) a history of such problems and a few simple tests can usually "rule out" these conditions.

In addition to determining that a patient is having a stroke, the initial goal of doctors is to determine which part of the brain is affected and what the exact cause of the stroke is. Unless the patient is in a coma, an experienced physician can usually determine what part of the brain is involved simply by performing a physical examination. Determining the cause of the stroke is not as simple, although the doctor can usually make an educated guess based on the stroke's location, the patient's history, and the frequency of the different causes of stroke (see Table 7.1). For example, if the stroke involves a part of the brain served by a single artery and the patient has a history of vascular disease, then an ischemic stroke caused by cerebrovascular disease is most likely.

When an ischemic stroke is suspected, the doctor must decide what part of the brain's circulation (see Fig. 2.1 on page 24) is involved in the stroke. In most cases the group of symptoms indicates exactly which artery is involved. For example, when a stroke results from obstruction of the carotid artery, the entire side of the body (on the side opposite the stroke) will be weak and numb. If only the anterior cerebral artery is involved, the leg is affected much more than the rest of the body, while if the middle cerebral artery is involved, the arm and face are affected more than the leg. If the vertebral or basilar arteries are involved, loss of coordination, vision problems, facial paralysis or numbness, and a variety of other problems can result. Depending on

Table 7.1 Incidence of the Various Types of Stroke

Type	Percentage of All Strokes
Ischemic strokes	85
Atherosclerosis	30
Emboli from heart to brain	25
Cause never determined	25
Emboli from other than heart	5
Hemorrhagic strokes*	15
Intracerebral hemorrhage	10
Subarachnoid hemorrhage	5

*The majority of intracerebral hemorrhage is caused by high blood pressure while most subarachnoid hemorrhage results from aneurysm.

just what areas are affected, an experienced neurologist can pinpoint the location of the stroke almost exactly.

DEVASTATING STROKE AND COMA

Most people remain awake and conscious during a stroke. When stroke is caused by hemorrhage, however, loss of consciousness is more likely. Ischemic strokes that involve the brain stem or the thalamus may also cause altered consciousness. No matter the cause, loss of consciousness following a stroke generally means it has involved critical parts of the brain. Persons who lose consciousness are less likely to recover from their stroke although this doesn't mean the situation is hopeless. Many people do recover completely after a long period of unconsciousness.

"Coma" is not a medical term with a clear definition (it's really more of a television medical show term). Usually it is used to mean that a person has remained unconscious and cannot be aroused by stimulation—even pain—for hours or days. Since there are many causes of coma—most of which aren't well understood—it is usually impossible for doctors to predict when a patient will regain consciousness.

WEAKNESS AND NUMBNESS

Weakness in one part of the body is a common symptom of stroke. Because the major motor functions arise in the cerebral cortex, a stroke involving any branch of the carotid artery will usually result in some degree of weakness on the opposite side of the body. The fiber tracts that leave the cortex travelling out to the body all pass through the brain stem, so strokes in this part of the brain can also result in paralysis.

Finding out exactly where the stroke has occurred will usually require determining what other symptoms are also present. For example, strokes in the cerebral cortex usually result in both loss of sensation and paralysis in the same area of the body. Strokes in the brain stem may result in partial paralysis or loss of coordination while sensation remains intact. Brain-stem strokes may also result in loss of some sensations while others remain intact. For example, a brain-stem stroke may result in loss of temperature sensation to part of the body, but the person can still feel a light touch or pressure in that area.

SPEECH AND HEARING DISORDERS

Loss of hearing can occur if the stroke involves the brain stem or the area of the temporal lobe that processes hearing. Strokes that involve the middle cerebral artery of the dominant (usually left) hemisphere can affect the ability to understand speech even though hearing may not be affected. Because the area of the brain that controls these functions is called Wernicke's area (after the person who discovered its function), this inability to understand speech is known as Wernicke's aphasia, from the Greek word meaning inability to speak.

Similarly, strokes of the same artery may affect Broca's area—the part of the brain that tells the mouth and throat how to form words.

In this case the person may understand speech perfectly well, but be unable to form words. In most cases, however, they can write perfectly well, unless there is also paralysis of the arm. Of course, this type of aphasia is called Broca's aphasia. Less commonly, the areas of the brain involved in recognizing written words are affected. Persons with strokes involving these areas may speak and understand speech perfectly well, but can no longer read or write.

While not strictly affecting speech, strokes in the brain stem often affect the muscles of the tongue, throat, and neck. This can make speech difficult to understand at first, but people affected in this way usually learn to speak coherently after rehabilitation. They often have a lot of difficulty swallowing, however, and may have trouble with choking when eating.

CHANGES IN MENTAL ABILITIES AND MEMORY

Because other symptoms, such as paralysis, are so frightening, it may be months after a stroke before changes involving memory or thinking become apparent. Almost any type of stroke can affect memory, although it is more common when the stroke has affected the temporal lobes of the cerebral cortex or structures near the thalamus.

Some strokes affect the ability to perform specific types of thinking. Strokes affecting the nondominant hemisphere (usually the right) are often likely to cause such problems. Some people are unable to add or subtract or can't recognize simple geometric shapes after this kind of stroke. Some can't recognize music. A person suffering such a stroke senses music no differently than random noise. In a few cases, the deficits are truly bizarre. Following a stroke involving the parietal lobe of the brain, for example, a person may not recognize that certain parts of their body actually belong to them. In the most dramatic cases, people affected in this way may insist that their left arm is not a part of their body.

Finally, many strokes affect emotion to some degree. In extreme cases, this may result in a dramatic inability to control emotion—fits of rage or sudden episodes of sobbing that occur for no reason. More commonly, the stroke victim simply becomes depressed. It is uncertain, however, how much of this depression results directly from brain damage caused by the stroke and how much is a normal result of the loss of abilities and functions that the stroke victim has suffered. Some rare strokes involving the frontal lobes cause people to become unable to recognize the emotions of others—they are incapable of recognizing when someone is angry, sad, or happy.

Medical Diagnosis of Stroke

The most important thing for a doctor to determine immediately following a stroke is whether the stroke was caused by ischemia (blocking of a blood vessel) or hemorrhage (bleeding). This is of critical importance because the treatment used for an ischemic stroke will worsen the effects of a hemorrhagic stroke.

CT SCAN AND MRI SCAN

The first test ordered once a stroke is suspected is either a CT or MRI scan of the brain. Although an MRI will provide more information regarding an ischemic stroke, it usually takes longer to schedule and perform than a CT scan. It also is more difficult for doctors and nurses to monitor a patient inside the MRI scanner, which may prove critically important.

No matter which scan is used, its purpose during the initial evaluation of a stroke is simply to determine if the stroke was caused by hemorrhage. Either type of scan can usually find an intracerebral hemorrhage quite accurately and can find a subarachnoid hemorrhage with only slightly less accuracy. If doctors still suspect a subarachnoid hemorrhage despite a normal scan, they will usually perform a lumbar puncture (see chapter 4) to determine if there is blood in the spinal fluid.

If an intracerebral hemorrhage is found, doctors will usually treat the patient's high blood pressure and give supportive care. If they suspect the bleeding was caused by an arteriovenous malformation, they may perform MRA (magnetic resonance angiography) or standard angiography, both of which are described in chapter 4. If a subarachnoid hemorrhage is found, angiography must be performed to determine the location and cause of bleeding.

If the stroke is ischemic, a CT scan will appear normal for at least twenty-four hours after the stroke, since the brain tissue remains intact at first, even though the cells have died. An MRI scan will sometimes show an ischemic stroke within four hours after it occurs, but may appear normal for twelve hours or more. For these reasons, the initial diagnosis of ischemic stroke is made when the patient exhibits the physical signs of a stroke and no evidence of hemorrhage is found on either an MRI or CT scan.

Once treatment of the ischemic stroke is begun, more tests will be ordered to determine exactly which artery the stroke originated from. If the symptoms involve the carotid artery and its branches, the initial tests will focus on that area. If the vertebral or basilar arteries are involved, vascular tests may not be performed until later, since there is no surgical treatment for problems in this area. If the patient's history makes it likely that an embolus caused the stroke, additional tests to evaluate the heart and other possible sources of the embolus may be needed.

ARTERIOGRAPHY AND OTHER TESTS OF THE BLOOD VESSELS

The preliminary tests will determine if the patient is having a stroke and can usually indicate whether the stroke is ischemic or hemorrhagic. If the stroke is caused by hemorrhage resulting from high blood pressure, further tests may not be necessary. Most other types of stroke will require further testing to determine exactly what the cause of the stroke was, however.

If the doctors are at all suspicious that the stroke may have been caused by atherosclerosis in the carotid arteries, they will usually order a special type of ultrasound study called duplex doppler. This type of ultrasound not only provides a picture of the blood vessel, it also determines how much blood is actually flowing through the vessel. The test is entirely painless and without complications. Because ultrasound waves do not pass through bone, the test cannot be used on the vertebral arteries or the branches of the carotid artery that lie within the skull.

If doctors are still concerned about the carotid artery, or if they are concerned about the vertebral and basilar arteries, they will usually perform digital subtraction angiography. This test involves injecting dye through an IV line and taking x-rays of blood vessels in the neck and base of the brain. When dye is injected into a vein, it must pass through the heart and lungs before reaching the arteries going to the brain and is therefore too diluted to be seen on standard x-rays. By using a digital computer to "subtract" all the other parts of the x-ray, however, a fairly clear picture of the larger arteries can be obtained. Since this test has fewer complications than a normal arteriogram, doctors prefer it if they don't need perfect images of the smaller arteries.

As an alternative, doctors may perform an MRA, or magnetic resonance angiogram. This test is exactly like having an MRI (see chapter 4), except that different dyes are used to show the arteries of the neck and brain. The test provides images that are similar in quality to those obtained with digital subtraction angiography, although they may provide a better picture of the arteries of the brain stem.

All these tests provide valuable information about the condition of the larger blood vessels leading to the brain. In many cases, however, more detailed information about these vessels or pictures of the smaller arteries within the brain may be needed. In this case angiography (sometimes called arteriography) will be necessary. Angiography will almost always be required to find the exact site of an aneurysm or arteriovenous malformation and may be necessary to find an atherosclerotic plaque in one of the smaller to medium-sized arteries of the brain.

As described in chapter 4, angiography requires a catheter to be inserted into a large artery of the groin or arm and threaded through the aorta to the large arteries going to the brain. The test can take several hours—it takes time to position the catheter and sometimes more than one artery will need to be studied. The images obtained by angiography are much more detailed and accurate than the ones obtained by the other types of vascular studies.

Angiography is safe (98 percent of people will have absolutely no problems from the study) but occasionally will cause complications. The most common complication is bleeding from the puncture site, which can usually be controlled by simple pressure. Less common is an allergic reaction to the injected dye or kidney problems as a result of the dye. In rare cases, angiography can worsen a stroke due to a catheter breaking off a small piece of atherosclerotic plaque, which becomes an embolus. Despite these rare complications, there is no substitute for the accurate images obtained by angiography. If these images are necessary, the patient really has no alternative but to take the test.

TESTS OF THE HEART AND BLOOD VESSELS

People who have suffered an embolic stroke will need to undergo diagnostic tests of their heart. This is necessary because the heart is the most common source of emboli—usually from blood clots that have formed around the heart valves or within the heart's chambers. Blood clots can form in the heart in a variety of conditions: after a heart attack, after heart surgery, if the atria (the smaller chambers of the heart) aren't contracting properly, if the heart valves are abnormal or have been replaced with artificial valves, or if the heart has become enlarged.

Unlike blood clots in other parts of the body, clots arising from the heart don't necessarily pass through the "screen" supplied by the lungs—they can travel directly to small arteries in the brain and cause a stroke. When one small piece of clot has broken off from a large blood clot in the heart, others are sure to follow if treatment isn't begun, so checking to be sure there is no blood clot in the heart is extremely important.

The test used to detect these clots is an ultrasound of the heart. This is a simple and painless test that will show any large clots in the heart and can also indicate if there are other existing problems that could potentially cause clots. In a few cases, an ultrasound or other study of the leg or other parts of the body may be done to determine that there are no clots in the veins.

If a stroke is found to be caused by atherosclerosis in the blood vessels of the brain, doctors will also suspect there is atherosclerosis in the vessels of the heart. Since this can lead to a heart attack, it may be necessary to perform a treadmill (stress) test or other tests to be certain that the stroke victim is not also at risk of a heart attack. These tests will usually not be done until after recovery from the stroke is well advanced, however.

CHAPTER 8

Treatment and Recovery Following a Stroke

The goal for all medical treatment of stroke is to keep as much brain tissue alive as possible. In a hemorrhagic stroke, this obviously means stopping the bleeding and preventing additional bleeding. While surgery may ultimately be necessary to accomplish this, medical treatment is usually the first line of defense when treating a hemorrhagic stroke.

Ischemic strokes are somewhat different. In most cases, the central area of brain tissue involved has absolutely no blood supply and will almost certainly die. In a few cases it may be possible to restore blood flow to this area quickly enough to save all the brain tissue involved, but this is not usually the case.

Around the central area (having no blood supply, however) is a region that has some blood supply, although not enough for neurons to function normally. In the areas closest to the center of the stroke, the blood supply may be sufficient to keep the neurons barely alive, but not sufficient to allow them to function. Since these neurons aren't functioning, under clinical examination they appear to be involved in the stroke. Nevertheless, they have the potential to return to full function if blood flow is improved.

Further away from the center of the stroke the neurons have enough blood supply to function normally, but if anything depletes their supply by even a small amount they may also stop functioning. If this occurs, the stroke becomes more severe and is called a progressive stroke. About 20 percent of all strokes become progressive.

The initial treatment of an ischemic stroke, therefore, consists of three efforts made at roughly the same time:

1. Support the patient to prevent complications. This may mean mechanical ventilation (a breathing machine) in severe strokes, or simply careful monitoring in less severe cases.
2. Restore blood flow to the affected area of the brain if that is at all possible.
3. Prevent any worsening of blood flow to nearby areas of the brain.

Overall, over 80 percent of persons having an ischemic stroke will survive. Of those who survive the first forty-eight hours following their stroke, more than 90 percent will survive. However, 30 percent of survivors will have another stroke within five years, although the risk can be dramatically lower for those who make significant changes to their lifestyle.

Persons having a hemorrhagic stroke have a lower survival rate (about 70 percent overall), but the survivors are less likely to have a long-term neurologic deficit (loss of brain function) than survivors of ischemic strokes. The survival rate and risk of suffering long-term problems vary a great deal depending upon the location and size of the hemorrhage, however.

Treatment of Ischemic Strokes

Even as the first diagnostic tests are being performed, the doctors treating a stroke victim will decide how much medical support is required. The initial medical support consists of making sure that the patient is breathing properly and that their blood pressure is acceptable. If the stroke involves areas of the brain that control respiration it may be necessary to use a mechanical ventilator (breathing machine) to breathe for the patient.

If the areas of the brain that control swallowing are affected, it may be necessary to take measures to prevent the patient from breathing saliva or other liquids into his or her lungs since this can result in severe pneumonia. Doctors may insert a tube through the nose to remove the contents of the stomach (called an NG, for naso-gastric tube), or they may insert a tube into the windpipe to prevent anything but air from entering the lungs. In the latter case, the patient is usually sedated and placed on a breathing machine.

Doctors will also make sure the patient's blood pressure is kept at the best level to provide blood to the brain. If blood pressure is too high or too low, medications will be given to restore it to an acceptable level. If blood pressure is difficult to control, doctors may also insert an arterial line, a catheter placed directly into the radial artery at the wrist. This allows them to monitor blood pressure more accurately than using a blood pressure cuff.

In some cases, medication to prevent blood clot formation will also be given. Whether the stroke was caused by an embolus, thrombus, or atherosclerotic plaque, preventing new blood clots from forming reduces the risk of the stroke enlarging or a second stroke from occurring. Of course, these medications can't be given until doctors are absolutely certain that the stroke is not caused by hemorrhage, so a CT or MRI scan will usually be performed before they are started.

Heparin has been used to prevent blood clot formation in stroke patients for many years, but there is still controversy over exactly which patients should receive it. Low molecular weight heparin— available for about ten years—may be safer because it is less likely to cause bleeding than regular heparin. Nevertheless, a large National Institutes of Health–sponsored study of low molecular weight heparin did not indicate any overall benefit to large numbers of stroke patients, although the drug was well tolerated. Heparin is still dictated by the individual patient's condition and the viewpoint of the treating physician.

IMMEDIATE TREATMENT TO REVERSE THE STROKE

One of the biggest advancements in stroke treatment has been the development of "clot-busting" drugs, medically referred to as thrombolytics (from thrombus, meaning clot, and lytic, meaning to dissolve). These drugs can actually dissolve blood clots that have already formed. This can, at least in theory, restore blood flow to areas of the brain that would otherwise die completely. It also can improve blood flow to areas near the stroke that have borderline blood flow.

Trials evaluating thrombolytics in patients with stroke have shown promising results if therapy is administered soon after symptom onset. The thrombolytic drug that currently is most widely used is called recombinant tissue plasminogen activator, mercifully abbreviated as rTPA or TPA by most doctors.

A large trial of thrombolytic treatment was conducted by the National Institute of Neurological Disorders and Stroke (NINDS) rTPA Stroke Study Group. All the patients in this study were treated within three hours of stroke onset. The study followed the patients for ninety days and found that TPA recipients had better outcomes; for example, they were 30 percent more likely to have no or only minimal disability than those who did not receive TPA. A second large study, the European Cooperative Acute Stroke Study (ECASS), gave TPA to persons within six hours of symptom onset. They, too, found benefit—although not as much as the NINDS study. They also found a higher rate of complication from the therapy.

The major complication from TPA therapy is bleeding. This may occur in any part of the body. For example, an ulcer or a several-days-old wound may begin bleeding after the therapy has begun. Since the blood vessels involved in a stroke can die just the same as neurons, restoring blood flow with TPA to an area of stroke could result in in-

CONTRAINDICATIONS TO RTPA USE IN ACUTE ISCHEMIC STROKE

- Intracranial hemorrhage, or previous intracranial hemorrhage
- More than three hours after onset of symptoms
- Previous stroke or serious head trauma within three months
- Rapidly improving or minor symptoms
- Symptoms suggestive of subarachnoid hemorrhage
- Major surgery within fourteen days
- Ulcer or other possible internal bleeding
- Seizure during the stroke
- Problems with blood clotting
- Use of oral anticoagulants or heparin within forty-eight hours
- Extremely high blood pressure at time of treatment

tracranial hemorrhage. In fact, this is a major complication of TPA therapy and represents the limiting factor for the use of these agents in stroke.

Most doctors now agree that TPA therapy should be attempted if it is certain an ischemic stroke is present and the symptoms are less than three hours old. Most also agree that if the symptoms are more than six hours old, the risk of intracranial hemorrhage is too high and the possible benefit too low to use TPA therapy. There are still differences of opinion regarding TPA therapy in strokes between three and six hours old, although several ongoing studies are attempting to clarify this problem. There are several contraindications to TPA therapy (see sidebar above), however, and patients with any of these contraindications are not candidates for this treatment no matter how soon they arrive at the hospital.

TPA is administered slowly through an IV and affects blood clots in all areas of the body. In a few cases, it is possible to administer TPA directly into the affected artery during an arteriogram. This permits smaller doses of the drug to be used since it is given exactly at the point where the stroke has occurred. Direct arterial injection allows some people to receive the drug who would otherwise be at too high a risk of bleeding. The procedure continues to be investigated, however, and it is uncertain if this technique is more beneficial than the standard technique.

MEDICATIONS TO PROTECT BRAIN CELLS

Over the last decade, research has revealed that some neurons can actually injure themselves when their blood supply is low. When the oxygen level becomes low, most neurons stop all activity to conserve their remaining oxygen. Some neurons become "overexcited" in the low oxygen conditions and send electrical signals even though they shouldn't. This activity causes them to use up the little oxygen they have remaining. The electrical signals from these excited neurons can also cause neighboring neurons to become excited, allowing the problem to spread.

Recent research has found several drugs that help prevent neurons from becoming overexcited when oxygen supplies are low. Many of these drugs work by blocking a receptor on neurons known as the NMDA receptor. Several of these NMDA antagonist medications are currently being used in Europe and Japan and are being studied in the U.S. A few are available for use here now, and more will be available by the time this book is published.

Some of these drugs (citicholine, lubelazole, tirilazad) have shown great promise in preliminary studies; they appear to be most effective in cases of evolving stroke. Patients who receive the medication have slightly better long-term outcomes and survival rates than patients who don't. Nimodipine, a different drug already available in the U.S., appears to provide protection in patients with certain types of subarachnoid hemorrhage, though its use in ischemic stroke has yielded mixed results.

THE FIRST FORTY-EIGHT HOURS AFTER STROKE

Once the initial treatments have begun, medical therapy focuses on preventing complications and preventing any extension of the stroke into areas of borderline blood flow. In many cases, the therapy consists of nothing more than carefully monitoring the patient for complications. This is of the utmost importance because complications occur in up to one-third of stroke victims.

A dedicated inpatient stroke unit is probably the safest place for a patient during the initial forty-eight hours following a stroke. Nurses are trained to recognize the earliest signs of complications, allowing immediate treatment of the problem. Monitoring in one of these intensive care units reduces the mortality rate following stroke and increases the proportion of patients with good outcomes.

Brain Swelling and Stroke Extension

The most common cause of death in the first seventy-two hours following stroke is swelling of the brain, or cerebral edema. Cerebral edema usually begins within twenty-four hours after the stroke's onset and may continue to worsen for ninety-six hours. The signs of cerebral edema usually include a decreased level of consciousness, worsening of existing neurological deficits, or development of new neurologic problems. The risk of cerebral edema correlates directly to the size of the stroke—people who suffer large strokes are much more likely to develop this complication.

When cerebral edema occurs, it further reduces blood flow to the brain, causing areas of borderline circulation to become areas of no circulation. This enlarges the area of the stroke and will add further to the amount of cerebral edema. This is one way in which a progressive stroke develops, with a cycle of swelling that causes more neurons to die, resulting in even more swelling.

If the edema becomes severe enough to involve an entire lobe of the brain, it may cause the brain to shift from its normal position in the skull. This is known as cerebral herniation (in the broadest sense, a hernia is any structure in the body that abnormally leaves its location). Cerebral herniation can crush the remaining healthy parts of the brain, usually resulting in death.

It should be apparent by now that one of the primary goals of early stroke treatment is preventing cerebral edema, or at least minimizing it should it occur. In every stroke patient, some measures are taken to minimize the chance of cerebral edema. If the stroke was small (and therefore the likelihood of cerebral edema is low), prevention may consist of little more than restricting fluid intake and careful monitoring to make sure the stroke's symptoms don't become worse.

For people experiencing large strokes, more aggressive measures are taken. This usually involves giving diuretics (fluid-removing medication) and strictly limiting the amount of fluid the patient receives. In many cases, this is enough to lower the pressure caused by cerebral edema and allow the body to begin to heal itself.

In more severe cases, the patient must be placed on a breathing machine and hyperventilation (breathing more rapidly than normal) performed. Hyperventilation removes carbon dioxide from the blood. When carbon dioxide levels are lowered, blood vessels in the brain will constrict, thus reducing the amount of swelling in the brain. Luckily, blood vessels that are damaged by atherosclerosis don't constrict very much when this is done so blood flow to areas near the stroke is not compromised by hyperventilation.

Whenever cerebral edema becomes this severe, doctors may place a monitor to actually measure pressure in the brain. Several types of monitors are available, but almost all require drilling a tiny hole in the skull under local anesthesia and placing a pressure monitor inside the skull. This gives doctors an accurate measurement of the actual pressure in the brain and tells them which therapy is working best to lower pressure.

In a very few cases of severe cerebral edema, doctors may actually remove part of the skull to provide additional space for the damaged brain to swell. In certain patients this procedure can be lifesaving, but it is used only as a last resort.

Other events that can cause stroke extension involve additional emboli that have reached the brain, or a clot that has enlarged and further blocked an artery. The risk of progressive stroke is greatest for patients with large strokes, those with embolic strokes arising from blood clots in the heart, and those with severe carotid artery atherosclerosis.

Treatment of this type of progressive stroke usually consists of increasing anticoagulant medication, but in a few cases emergency surgery to remove carotid plaque or even a blood clot from the heart may be indicated. Patients with large strokes who are given anticoagulants have increased risk of cerebral hemorrhage, however, so this therapy is not without risk.

The final reason for progressive stroke is hemorrhagic transformation. Hemorrhagic transformation of a stroke occurs when blood vessels in the area of the original ischemic stroke break down. If some blood flow has been restored to the area, bleeding can result. Hemorrhagic transformation occurs in as many as 20 percent of patients with ischemic stroke, although it is often small and causes no problem. Embolic strokes are more likely to be associated with hemorrhagic transformation because the embolus eventually dissolves allowing blood flow to return to the area.

Medical Treatment and Support

In addition to treatment of the stroke itself, constant attention must be given to preventing medical complications that can develop following a stroke. Most stroke victims also have other medical conditions—such as heart disease or diabetes—that may worsen during the stress of the stroke. Medical complications involving organs other than the brain occur in as many as 30 percent of stroke patients, and preventing them, or at least treating them rapidly once they have occurred, is the key to a good outcome.

Because preventing complications is so important, every bit of information you can supply to the medical team helps to improve the odds of a good outcome. A medical history will usually be taken from family members, but often you will remember things hours later—a drug allergy, a family history of a certain medical problem, etc. If that happens, be sure to tell one of the nurses as soon as you recall the information. It could be the key to preventing an unnecessary complication.

Intensive Care and Ventilation   As discussed earlier, mechanical ventilation may be needed if the breathing or swallowing centers of the brain are affected, or if hyperventilation is needed to control cerebral edema. In most cases, if mechanical ventilation is needed in the early phase following a stroke, it will be continued for at least three to five days, since this is the period needed for cerebral edema to decrease and brain function to return.

In a few cases, ventilation (or at least a breathing tube) may even be required for a period of several weeks. Although this is obviously not a good situation, it does not mean the patient is hopeless; many people recover significantly even after weeks of mechanical ventilation. It's also important for family members to realize that when a patient is mechanically ventilated, they are usually heavily sedated or even given medications to paralyze their muscles. This can be critically important to keep them from fighting against the ventilator, but will make it impossible for them to respond when a family member visits. In some cases, although the medication keeps the patient from responding, they can hear perfectly well. It is important that family members keep a positive attitude anytime they are in the room with the stroke patient.

In addition to maintaining breathing, many other body functions may need treatment during the period after a stroke. Often, the normal regulation of fluid balance in the body is upset either by direct damage to the brain or because of medications given to treat cerebral edema. Additionally, about 10 percent of persons suffering large strokes develop the "syndrome of inappropriate antidiuretic hormone," which is usually referred to simply as SIADH. In this condition, the brain abnormally secretes hormones telling the kidneys to conserve every drop of water. This can worsen cerebral edema and cause changes in the body's salt content.

If SIADH develops, doctors and nurses will take great care to calculate exactly how much fluid and salt the patient receives each day. It is extremely important not to "sneak" a soft drink, extra water, or a candy bar to the patient during this time. Doing so could cause major medical problems and even worsen the amount of brain damage.

Controlling Blood Pressure   Blood pressure is often elevated following a stroke. After an ischemic stroke, slightly higher blood pressure could help supply more blood to the brain, so doctors will not treat a mild elevation in blood pressure. Very high blood pressure can worsen cerebral edema or cause hemorrhage into the area of stroke, however. If blood pressure reaches this level, it will have to be treated.

Treating high blood pressure may only consist of giving medications by mouth. In more severe cases, or if cerebral edema is also present, blood pressure medications are given through an intravenous line. In this case an arterial line will probably be inserted into the small artery at the wrist to monitor the blood pressure.

Treatment of Hemorrhagic Strokes

Most of the general treatments described for patients with ischemic strokes (intensive care monitoring, treating cerebral edema, preventing complications, etc.) also apply to patients who have had hemorrhagic strokes. Instead of considering medications to prevent blood clotting, however, treatments that will stop bleeding—or at least prevent it from restarting—will be undertaken.

The main method for reducing bleeding following a hemorrhagic stroke is giving medications to reduce blood pressure to slightly lower than normal levels. The head of the bed will usually be elevated (this will lower blood pressure to the brain slightly), and the patient will often be sedated to minimize anxiety and control pain. Bleeding will also be monitored by checking the patient's neurologic status every hour or two and (usually) repeating a CT or MRI scan every day or two.

SUBARACHNOID HEMORRHAGE

If the bleeding is subarachnoid (outside the brain), the problem usually doesn't affect one specific part of the brain and therefore doesn't cause a focal (affecting only one part of the body) deficit. Instead, patients are likely to have a severe headache and a reduced level of consciousness. If loss of consciousness occurs, the patient may require mechanical ventilation. If the bleeding is severe enough to increase the pressure around the brain, a pressure monitor as described above may be inserted.

Subarachnoid hemorrhage is associated with a specific complication known as cerebral vasospasm. Cerebral vasospasm is very tight contraction (spasm) of arteries near the site of bleeding. The spasm can completely cut off blood supply to areas of the brain causing an ischemic stroke to develop. It occurs in as many as 30 percent of people following a subarachnoid hemorrhage, but in most cases its effects aren't extremely severe. It is most likely to happen from three to five days following the hemorrhage, but may occur as much as ten days later.

In most cases, doctors will give medication (nimodipine or nicardipine are frequently used) to help prevent cerebral vasospasm. They will also carefully monitor the patient's fluid status because dehydration can trigger cerebral vasospasm. Finally, doctors will usually delay surgery to repair an aneurysm or other bleeding problem for a few weeks if possible since vasospasm is more likely to occur following surgery.

INTRACEREBRAL HEMORRHAGE

Persons with intracerebral hemorrhage are treated differently than those with subarachnoid hemorrhage. Because they are less likely to develop cerebral vasospasm and more likely to have high blood pressure, patients will almost always be given medications to lower their blood pressure. Because the bleeding actually tears and compresses specific parts of the brain near the bleeding site, they are also more likely to have focal neurologic deficits.

Depending upon the actual location in the brain and the amount of hemorrhage that has occurred, the deficits may be minimal or quite severe. If the hemorrhage is large and involves the brain stem, it is very likely to be fatal no matter what treatment is used. Small hemorrhages that don't involve the brain stem generally have a good outcome when treated with blood pressure reducing medications and careful monitoring. In either case, surgery is not likely to benefit the condition. Surgery may be indicated, however, if the intracerebral hemorrhage resulted from an aneurysm or arteriovenous malformation within the brain.

SURGERY FOR HEMORRHAGIC STROKE

While emergency surgery is almost never indicated for ischemic stroke, it is sometimes required for hemorrhagic stroke. However, medical studies have shown that persons with hemorrhagic stroke who suffer complete loss of consciousness, heart disturbances, or develop extremely high pressure within the brain generally do not benefit from surgery.

Surgery will eventually be needed for most patients who suffer subarachnoid hemorrhage from an aneurysm or arteriovenous malformation. In general, doctors will wait several weeks before performing the surgery since this lowers the risk of cerebral vasospasm. In some cases, the risk of further bleeding is greater than the risk of vasospasm, however, and surgery will be performed within a day or two of the subarachnoid hemorrhage.

Whether it's performed as an emergency procedure or electively after several weeks, the surgery basically consists of placing a metal clip across the base of the aneurysm so that blood cannot leak from the weakened aneurysm wall. The actual risks of the surgery depend upon exactly where the aneurysm is located and will be explained in detail by the neurosurgeon beforehand.

In a few cases of intracerebral hemorrhage, surgery may be considered. Usually, these involve patients who have a fairly large hemorrhage that does not involve the brain stem (large hemorrhages in the brain stem are invariably fatal). The purpose of the surgery is to drain the blood out of the brain so that it doesn't crush or tear nearby brain tissue. The actual procedure almost always successfully removes the blood from the brain. The individual patient's outcome following surgery is quite variable, however, and doctors probably won't be able to predict how much brain function will be regained until several days later.

Initial Recovery in the Hospital

Once the risks of cerebral edema, extension of the stroke, or further hemorrhage have passed, the patient is considered to be stable. The stabilization period following a stroke can take as little as two days, or as long as several weeks depending upon the severity and type of stroke suffered. Once the patient is considered stable, they can be moved out of the stroke care unit to a regular hospital room for early rehabilitation.

That doesn't mean that all risks are over. Stroke patients remain at risk of developing complications for weeks or even months. After the first forty-eight hours has passed, any life-threatening consequences usually involve complications rather than the stroke itself. The patient must still be watched carefully to identify any complications as soon as possible so that treatment begins as rapidly as possible.

COMMON COMPLICATIONS FOLLOWING STROKE

Fever

Nearly half of all patients with stroke will develop a fever. In some cases it is caused by damage to the temperature control centers of the brain. More commonly, the fever develops for an obvious reason: an infection has developed somewhere in the body. In any case, the fever must be controlled because an elevated temperature can worsen the amount and severity of brain injury. Treatment will typically include medications, such as Tylenol® or aspirin, but may require alcohol baths or even ice bags.

At the same time, doctors will take blood samples and perform other tests to make sure there is no infection. Attention will focus on the lungs and urinary tract since pneumonia and bladder infections are common during recovery from stroke.

Dysphagia

Dysphagia means difficulty swallowing. About one-third of patients will develop dysphagia following a stroke. The risk is higher if the stroke involves the brain stem and lower if it only involves the cerebral cortex. In some cases the dysphagia is obvious when the patient tries to eat or drink, but in others it may not be apparent at all. Because persons with dysphagia are at risk for aspiration (food or liquids entering the lungs, which can cause pneumonia), all patients who've had a stroke should be tested to make sure they can swallow normally.

If dysphagia does occur, it may be necessary to insert a tube into the stomach to provide food and liquids. In most cases rehabilitation can retrain the swallowing muscles over a period of weeks, but in a few cases a permanent feeding tube may be necessary.

Pneumonia

Pneumonia is the most common and feared complication after a stroke; it causes 25 percent of all stroke-related deaths. Pneumonia tends to develop in older patients whose immune systems are weakened and in bedridden patients who have dysphagia because they can inhale saliva and food into their lungs.

Although most of us think pneumonia is treated easily with antibiotics, this isn't the case for stroke patients for several reasons. First, pneumonia is much more difficult to treat in patients who are bedridden or who can't cough properly because of paralysis. Second, if aspiration from dysphagia occurs, the patient may have repeated bouts of pneumonia. Finally, hospital bacteria are more likely to be resistant to antibiotics, so most of the commonly used antibiotics are not effective against "hospital-acquired" pneumonia.

Deep Vein Thrombosis

Deep vein thrombosis (DVT) occurs when blood remains in the leg veins until it forms blood clots inside the veins. The clots may break off and travel to the lungs where they can cause a pulmonary embolism—blocking of the lung's circulation by the clot. If the embolus is very large it can cause death by blocking all the lung's circulation. Even smaller emboli can lower the oxygen content of the blood (especially if pneumonia is also present) by blocking some circulation to the lungs. They can also cause heartbeat irregularities.

The primary prevention of DVT is movement of the legs, especially by walking, which prevents blood from pooling in the veins. For this reason, doctors will make every effort to have patients walking as soon as possible after a stroke. If walking is impossible, physical therapists will move and massage the patient's legs to help prevent thrombosis. Additionally, the patient will have to wear elastic stockings to "squeeze" blood out of the leg veins. Doctors may also start medications to prevent blood clots from forming.

If DVT does occur, it is considered a medical emergency because it leads to fatal pulmonary embolism in approximately 10 percent of patients. In such cases, high doses of anticoagulant medications will be given since the risk of pulmonary embolus is greater than the risk of hemorrhage. In rare cases, surgery may be performed to insert a filter into the vena cava (the large vein leading back to the heart) to prevent emboli from reaching the lungs.

Urinary Tract Infection

Urinary infections following stroke are most likely when the patient requires a urinary catheter to help empty their bladder. They may also occur if the bladder doesn't empty completely, remaining partially filled with urine at all times. Urinary infections are generally less severe than pneumonia, however, and are effectively treated with antibiotics in most cases.

Seizures

About 5 to 10 percent of stroke patients will eventually develop seizures. Seizures result when an area of the brain was damaged, but not completely destroyed, by the stroke. This area can send out abnormal electrical impulses that "recruit" other brain cells, eventually causing large portions of the brain to send out random messages, resulting in a seizure.

Seizures that occur during the first twenty-four hours after a stroke are considered a sign of severe brain damage. Seizures developing after the initial twenty-four hours do not necessarily indicate severe damage, however. In fact, the eventual outcome for patients who develop seizures more than twenty-four hours after a stroke is no worse than for those who never have seizures.

The risk of developing seizures is not just limited to the period immediately following the stroke. Only one-third of stroke patients who eventually develop seizures will actually have a seizure within the first two weeks of recovery. The most common time to develop a seizure is between the fourth and tenth weeks after the stroke.

Seizures are more likely when a large ischemic stroke involving the cerebral hemisphere has occurred. They are also likely in patients who've suffered an intracerebral hemorrhage. Anticonvulsant medication will control the seizures in almost every case. In some cases, anticonvulsants can be stopped within a year after the stroke, but some people will require them for the rest of their lives.

REHABILITATION

Rehabilitation following a stroke is a difficult, time-consuming process. It usually begins in the hospital within days of the stroke and then continues in a rehabilitation hospital or outpatient facility. During the first days after a stroke, a physical therapist may work alone performing range of motion exercises or helping the patient walk. Once the stroke victim has stabilized, an entire rehabilitation team becomes involved. The team includes nurses, physical therapists, social workers, and speech therapists, all working under the direction of a physician specializing in stroke rehabilitation.

In order for rehabilitation to be successful, the patient must cooperate with the therapists. While this may seem obvious, the most common reason for "failed" rehabilitation is a patient who is not willing to perform the work needed. The rehabilitation process may take several months, during which patients may become severely depressed or may not believe that any improvement is possible after their stroke. The reality is that most people can regain a lot of function and restore lost abilities following even a very large stroke.

Overall, about 75 percent of patients who survive their stroke will improve markedly during a rehabilitation program, and the average length of the intensive portion of the program (more than three sessions a week) is about thirty days. This is usually followed by a less intensive program (two or less sessions per week) lasting several months. Overall, two-thirds of stroke victims are able to return to a completely independent lifestyle following rehabilitation, and less than 10 percent require long-term care.

Physical and Occupational Therapy

Early physical therapy may consist of the therapist moving paralyzed portions of the body to prevent wasting and shortening of muscles. They will also provide padding and pillows to prevent decubitus ulcers (bedsores) from developing and make special splints to prevent contractures (permanent shortening of muscles). Within a day or two, therapists will try to have the patient sitting up in a bedside chair and walking with assistance if possible.

Physical therapists will begin exercising weakened muscle groups within a week after the stroke. At the same time, occupational therapists will fit special braces to provide as much support and function as possible. These may involve placing a brace on a weakened leg so that walking becomes possible, or designing a special splint to hold a weakened hand in a useful position. Social workers assist the therapists by helping the patient access government services or insurance benefits to pay for wheelchairs, braces, and other necessary equipment.

A major focus of physical therapy is on walking because strokes that affect muscles, balance, or coordination can all interfere with the ability to walk. If walking isn't possible, therapy may focus on being able to move from bed to wheelchair unassisted so that the patient can move about as they wish. Secondary goals will involve restoring function to hands affected by the stroke, or training the patient to do tasks with the opposite hand.

Before the patient returns home, the therapists will usually meet with family members to help them obtain any needed equipment. A huge variety of devices ranging from shower chairs to walkers to special beds and reclining chairs are available to make home life easier for patients experiencing problems with strength or balance following their stroke.

The rehabilitation team should also introduce both the patient and family to stroke support groups in their area. Support groups not only provide emotional and educational support, they can often arrange discounts for equipment and services for stroke patients. There are also many national and regional support groups, as well as groups with Internet sites (see appendix B).

Speech Therapy

About 20 percent of stroke victims will experience some form of difficulty with communication. This may involve problems speaking, understanding speech, reading, writing, or even remembering conversations. Persons who suffer these problems often say communication problems are far more frustrating for them than paralysis.

Happily, a variety of techniques have been developed that allow patients to either regain the ability to speak and understand, or develop alternative methods of communication. In many cases, the family must be actively involved in this therapy since it is particularly important that they learn how to communicate with the stroke victim.

Speech therapists may also work with those victims who have dysphagia (difficulty swallowing) as a result of their stroke. In many cases, they can help the patient relearn how to swallow and protect themselves from aspiration.

Other Services

Most stroke rehabilitation teams have other specialists available as consultants. The team may suggest evaluation by a psychologist, involvement of a chaplain, or any of several other individuals. It is important that both family and patient take an active role in asking for the help they need. Therapists are not particularly adept at mind reading, and any problem can be compounded when a patient is too embarrassed to admit they are depressed, afraid, or simply can't afford certain items needed for rehabilitation.

CHAPTER 9

Long-Term Outcome After Stroke

How Long Can You Continue to Improve?

The length of time it takes for rehabilitation to restore maximum function varies from patient to patient, but certain functions return more quickly than others. Motor (movement) functions are usually the quickest to recover while complex functions, such as speech, may take quite a bit longer.

Areas of the body that are completely paralyzed following a stroke will usually not recover to any great degree. Areas of weakness can improve rapidly in strength during the first month after a stroke, and improvement in strength and mobility is usually complete within six months. In general, movement and function of the leg recover more completely compared to the arm.

While overall movement and strength may be maximally improved within six months, more coordinated movements, such as walking or performing complex tasks with the hand, can continue to improve for up to two years following a stroke. To some extent, this delay results because it is impossible to start rehabilitation of more complicated, coordinated movements until strength and motion have been restored. Additionally, these movements require several areas of the brain to work together, and recovery of such activities generally takes longer than simple tasks involving just one area of the brain.

Difficulty swallowing will usually improve to some degree over the first two months after a stroke, as will double vision and other problems involving the eye muscles. In most cases, these problems will improve to their maximum extent within six months following the stroke. At this point doctors may want to consider surgery to correct weakened eye muscles or other measures to aid eating and drinking.

Other functions return more slowly than motor functions. Communication problems often improve very slowly at first, but patients can continue to make progress in these areas for two or more years following a stroke. Similarly, problems with memory, thought processes, or emotional stability will often improve slowly for several years following a stroke.

Learning to Live with a Stroke's Effects

As recovery following stroke progresses, it will become apparent which physical and mental problems will resolve with continued therapy and which ones won't. The second goal of stroke rehabilitation is to learn how to cope with the remaining problems.

WEAKNESS AND PARALYSIS

Despite aggressive therapy, most stroke victims are left with at least some areas of minor weakness—if not complete paralysis. In many cases, using braces or assisting devices will allow the patient to walk and perform almost all the normal tasks of everyday life. In others, a wheelchair may be necessary but even then simple adjustments in the home can allow the stroke victim to be self-sufficient in most cases.

Weakness may be compounded by dizziness or loss of coordination, which will increase the likelihood of falling. For this reason it is important to be certain that canes, walkers, or other assisting devices are available and used. Falls remain the most common source of further injury in persons who have had a stroke.

Areas of complete muscle paralysis are likely to develop spasticity over the weeks and months following a stroke. Spasticity is muscle shortening and rigidity that occurs because of abnormal nerve input into the muscles. If untreated, spasticity will eventually lead to contractures, a permanent shortening of the muscles that leaves the joint in a fixed position.

Soon after a stroke, therapists will begin stretching muscles, moving extremities, and even fitting splints to prevent spasticity and contractures from occurring. It may be necessary for the patient to continue using splints at home and for family members or therapists to continue to move the affected limbs for months or years after the stroke. If spasticity becomes severe or causes pain, doctors can prescribe medications that will reduce it. Most of these medications cause drowsiness and other side effects, at first, but these will often clear up within a few weeks.

NUMBNESS, ABNORMAL SENSATION, AND PAIN

Most stroke patients experience altered sensations in some part of their body. Complete loss of sensation is uncommon; usually there is loss of certain sensations and sparing of others. For example, a person may be able to tell when something touches their arm, but could not determine if the object is hot or cold.

Sometimes certain sensations become abnormally uncomfortable after a stroke. The affected area may be overly sensitive to cold, or a light touch may be perceived as uncomfortable. Additionally, the pain regulating areas of the brain may be affected so that minor pain becomes almost unbearable. For example, the aching pain from an arthritic shoulder may become much more severe after a stroke involving that arm. If the area affected by the stroke is also paralyzed, it may become swollen because blood will tend to pool in that area. Swelling can also become painful, adding to the patient's discomfort.

Any abnormal painful sensations following a stroke will usually decrease over the first six months, although they may not disappear entirely. In almost every case, however, the pain can be treated effectively. Swelling can be reduced by wearing elastic gloves or stockings, and hypersensitivity can be reduced by physical therapy. Medications will generally control any remaining pain. Interestingly, standard pain medications are often not very effective in controlling post-stroke pain. Doctors often find that anti-inflammatory medications and certain antiseizure medications control this pain better than narcotics and other pain pills.

Two particularly painful conditions affect some people after a stroke. Shoulder-hand syndrome occurs in about 10 percent of people who have a stroke causing paralysis of the arm. The patient with shoulder-hand syndrome often has incredible hypersensitivity of the arm and hand—even a breeze blowing across the area or sheets rubbing against it are painful. The arm is usually quite swollen and often becomes reddened.

Shoulder-hand syndrome may require nerve blocks (injections of local anesthetics near the nerves) or other therapies to control the pain and should usually be treated by a pain specialist. An orthopedic specialist should also be involved since chronic dislocation of the shoulder frequently occurs in people with paralysis of the arm. This can cause many of the same symptoms.

The second painful condition is known as post-thalamic infarct pain. This problem occurs when the stroke has involved that part of the thalamus that processes sensations. Among its other functions, this part of the brain processes signals coming from the body and sends them to the proper parts of the cerebral cortex for processing. Patients whose stroke involves the thalamus typically develop widespread pains that often involve large areas of the body. The pain is difficult to describe: it may include sensations such as burning, aching, and hypersensitivity, but these are not always present. Although certain medications can reduce this pain, the condition is difficult to treat.

MENTAL AND MEMORY DEFICITS

Almost two-thirds of stroke patients report that they have some type of mental impairment following their stroke. This may be quite obvious, such as when someone has trouble communicating, but these difficulties can range from a bit of forgetfulness to complete dementia (a medical term meaning loss of contact with reality). Luckily, the mental deficits are mild in most cases.

Most stroke patients find their long-term memory is intact; they have no problem recognizing family members or remembering events that occurred months or years before. Many have problems with short-term memory, however. This may be the simple forgetfulness that occurs in many people when they are stressed, or it may be more severe and cause extreme difficulty in remembering phone numbers, tasks that they planned to perform, or even what they were about to say.

Thought problems may be specific (the problem may only involve using numbers, or trying to read a map) or can involve all forms of thinking. Thinking difficulties may be so severe that decision making is impaired in almost all areas of life. Or it may simply be a source of frustration to the stroke victim that goes unnoticed by others.

In most cases, memory and thought difficulties improve rapidly over the first six months following a stroke and continue to improve slowly for another year or two. Psychologists can perform a battery of tests that will indicate exactly what types of problems the patient has and can suggest coping strategies that will help the person deal with them effectively.

Simple commonsense adjustments can help, particularly with memory problems. Many stroke sufferers find they can cope with memory deficits by keeping lists and writing down what they planned to do. Obviously, this is not possible for stroke victims who cannot write, but many simple-to-operate pocket voice recorders can perform the same function. Family members can also help by being careful not to interrupt when the stroke sufferer is speaking, by making lists for them, and by developing a structured schedule that is easier for them to remember.

Thought process problems are more difficult to deal with, both because they may be less apparent and because the person suffering from them usually goes to some lengths to deny their existence. If family members are concerned, they should ask for testing and other evaluations to determine exactly how severe the problem is. In some cases legal arrangements should be made to protect the patient's finances and property from possible lapses in judgment.

MOOD CHANGES AND DEPRESSION

Depression and mood changes occur in two-thirds of all stroke patients and in almost all patients with strokes that involve the frontal lobe on the left side. Emotional problems are severe in about one-third of stroke patients, at least during the first year. For most patients the mood change encompasses depression only, which is usually due to the situation, rather than being caused by direct brain damage. Antidepressant medication and either group or individual therapy are both helpful in such cases. Generally, situational depression will clear up within a year after the stroke, but some patients require antidepressants for a longer period of time.

If the stroke involves areas of the brain that help regulate emotions, then mood problems may be more severe and unusual. Sudden bursts of extreme emotion may occur involving spells of inappropriate laughter, crying fits, or bursts of anger. Again, medication is available that can help prevent these problems, although doctors often have to try two or three different medications to find the one that works for an individual patient. It is also important for friends and family members to realize that these episodes are neither their fault nor the stroke patient's fault.

In a few cases, the mood problems are more complex. Paranoia and even delusions may occur. A few patients develop obsessive-compulsive behavior, such as repeatedly washing their hands or sitting only in a certain location in a room. Such behaviors may occur only during times of stress, or may be constant. In either case, they usually respond well to medication. The doctor can only treat these problems if he or she knows about them, however. Sometimes family members hesitate to bring up such problems out of embarrassment or fear that the doctor won't understand. In reality, while these problems aren't common after a stroke, they occur often enough that a doctor will consider them a routine part of post-stroke care.

URINARY INCONTINENCE AND RETENTION

Bladder difficulties are not particularly common following a stroke but can be an annoying and embarrassing problem when they do occur. It is important that any stroke patient with urinary problems be checked carefully by a doctor to make sure there is no urinary infection present.

Incontinence (unexpected urination) is more common in women but can also occur in men. It may take any of several forms. Stress incontinence—which usually occurs in females—results if the muscles of the pelvis are weakened. In this situation anything that increases pressure on the bladder, such as coughing or sneezing, can cause urination since the muscles that hold the urethra closed are weakened. Medications are available that can help the problem, although some people will require absorbing undergarments (females) or a condom-type catheter (males).

Overflow incontinence results when the bladder doesn't empty well (called urinary retention). In this case, the bladder becomes so full that it eventually overflows, resulting in unexpected urination.

Urinary retention can also occur without incontinence. Urinary retention in males is often associated with prostate enlargement, which may require surgery. In females, and in males with normal prostates, retention is usually treated by teaching the patient to catheterize themselves (inserting a small, soft tube to drain the bladder) several times a day.

DRIVING

After rehabilitation, most stroke patients (and their families) want to know if they can drive. Usually, the decision depends more upon vision and mental abilities than on physical limitations. A variety of mechanical adaptations, such as hand throttles and brakes, and even vans designed for a wheelchair-bound driver, are available to allow most people to drive.

Problems with double or blurred vision, possible seizures, memory lapses, or sedation from medications are much more likely to limit the ability to drive than are physical problems. If none of these problems exist, driving is usually no problem. If there is a question about the patient's ability to drive, it is important for the patient and family to decide together if driving is safe and necessary. The decision should usually involve a discussion with the patient's physician, who will have knowledge of state regulations for handicapped drivers.

For Family Members

Family members must endure much emotional upheaval in the first weeks following a stroke. At first, there is the awful fear that their loved one may not even live through the stroke, followed by concern that another stroke may occur. Depending upon how severe the stroke is, the first weeks and even months after the stroke are filled with worrying about whether the stroke victim will be able to care for themselves, can return to live at home, and even if they'll "still be themselves" after the stroke.

During the recovery phase, even more will be asked of family members. Therapists may want you to come to speech and occupational therapy to better learn how to communicate with and help the person who has suffered the stroke. During the transition to assisted and then home living, you will be asked to help with everyday care: eating, bathing, even moving about may all require assistance at first. At the same time you may need to make major modifications to your home so that the stroke sufferer can function as independently as possible. And always there is the financial fear that accompany medical bills, lost income, and the need for special equipment at home.

This often becomes overwhelming, and it's not surprising that families of stroke victims often find themselves frustrated and depressed as the recovery process continues. Circumstances and stress are sometimes made even worse as the stroke victim, who is also afraid or depressed, makes more demands for help and companionship from his family.

It is important to remember what the airline pilot says just before take off: "In case of emergency put your own oxygen mask on first, then assist others." Recovery from stroke is a long process. If you don't take care of yourself first, soon you won't be able to take care of anyone else. You may feel guilty about going to a movie or spending a day with your grandchildren while your spouse is in physical therapy. If you don't do some things for your own enjoyment, however, it's only a matter of time until you become depressed, exhausted, and resentful.

Remember also to monitor your own physical and emotional health carefully. For spouses and children of a stroke victim, the recovery period is a time of high stress. You are more likely to suffer physical illness (or worsening of an existing illness), anxiety attacks, and depression during this time. If you do become depressed or

anxious, see your doctor. Temporary use of an antidepressant or antianxiety medication can help you to avoid needless suffering.

At the same time, the encouragement and support of family members has been shown to be of great benefit to the stroke victim. It has
been shown that for people who suffer strokes of similar severity,
those with positive family support will have better outcomes than
those without such support. Positive support, however, doesn't mean
tons of sympathy and waiting on the stroke victim hand and foot. This
does not encourage the stroke sufferer to get better or to learn to
function independently. Rather, an attitude of positive support means
providing help that is absolutely necessary and making adjustments to
allow the stroke victim to care for herself as much as possible.

For example, lowering a sink and installing bath railings and a
shower chair so that stroke sufferers can bathe themselves is much
more encouraging than giving them a bath. Similarly, making arrangements so that they can cook for themselves is much better than
having meals brought in three times a day. In the long run, these kinds
of adjustments will allow stroke sufferers to still feel useful and a part
of the family, rather than a burden.

There are a lot of resources available to help you. In the hospital,
social workers and therapists can put you in contact with many agencies available to help ease the stress. There are stroke recovery and
support groups in most major cities (see appendix B), and government
and volunteer agencies that can help with transportation, special
equipment, and even cooking and meals. When equipment must be
bought with your own funds, remember that used medical equipment
is just as functional as new equipment and can cost less than half as
much. The yellow pages usually list used medical equipment suppli-
ers who resell equipment or can arrange leases for equipment that
may only be needed temporarily.

PART III

Brain Tumors

CHAPTER 10

The Different
Types of
Brain Tumors

What Are Brain Tumors?

Possibly no diagnosis is more frightening than a brain tumor. It is extremely important to understand, however, that a brain tumor is not just one disease; it really includes dozens of different kinds of tumors, which have very different treatments and outcomes. Certain brain tumors are among the most easily cured of all tumors while others are impossible, at present, to treat effectively.

Brain tumors not only differ from each other, they are very different from tumors that occur in other parts of the body. When a tumor occurs elsewhere, whether it is malignant (possibly lethal) or benign (not lethal) depends only on the type of cells that the tumor contains. If the cells are the type that spread to other areas, the tumor may metastasize (give rise to other tumors in other locations) and is therefore considered potentially lethal. If the cells are not the type that spread, the tumor is not lethal and surgery can remove it completely.

In the brain, however, the type of cells a tumor contains is only one of the factors that determines if the tumor is potentially lethal. If the tumor contains metastasizing cells it will, of course, be malignant and may spread to other areas. Some brain tumors that do not spread are still potentially lethal, however, because they are located in an area of the brain from which the tumor cannot be removed. Although 44 percent of all primary brain tumors are considered benign as far as their cellular makeup, even a benign brain tumor may result in death.

Overall, brain tumors are not very common. There are only about 21,000 new cases of primary brain tumor (a tumor that started in the brain) diagnosed in the U.S. each year. Another 20,000 people are diagnosed with a secondary brain tumor (a tumor that originated in another part of the body, then spread to the brain). In 1995, primary brain tumors represented about 1.5 percent of all cancers diagnosed and 2 percent of cancer deaths.

Unfortunately, the cure rate for many types of brain tumors is significantly lower than the cure rate for most other types of cancer. Sadly, brain tumors are especially likely to affect the young. They are the second leading cause of cancer death in children under age fifteen and in young adults up to age thirty-four.

Currently, the causes of primary brain tumors are not known. Genetics does play some role, but exactly how important is not well understood. Environmental agents and other possibilities are under investigation.

Classifications of Brain Tumors

TUMOR TYPE

The classification of brain tumors is rather complex, especially considering there are several dozen different types of brain tumors. While there is no way to make brain tumor classification a simple subject, it is possible to explain it in understandable terms by placing the various types of brain tumors into related groups.

The first step in understanding tumor categories is to understand the names used to describe tumors. Tumors, no matter what part of the body they occur in, usually have a name that ends in *oma*, whether they are benign or malignant. The tumor's name also identifies the type of tissue that it originated from. Thus, the name *adenoma* means tumors arising from glandular tissue, while *carcinoma* is a tumor originating from the skin or tissue lining a body cavity, and *sarcoma* identifies a tumor as beginning in connective tissue (such as muscle or bone).

Secondary brain tumors (those originating in other parts of the body and metastasizing to the brain) are identified by the name of the original cancer preceded by the word *metastatic*. For example, if the secondary brain tumor originated from a lung cancer, it will be called a metastatic pulmonary carcinoma (a cancer originating from the cells lining the lungs).

Primary brain tumors (those originating from brain cells) generally follow the same naming rules that are used for other cancers. A primary tumor of the pituitary gland (see chapter 1) is called a pituitary adenoma, for instance. However, since the brain contains several unique tissues, such as supporting cells, a brain tumor is often classified by the exact type of tissue it originated from. Thus, a meningioma means a tumor originating from the meningeal membranes. A glioma arises from the glial cells (the supporting cells of the brain) such as astrocytes (see chapter 1). Some brain tumors are so primitive that they seem to have originated from cells that are only supposed to exist in the developing fetus, cells that should not exist in the adult brain at all. The term *blastoma* is used to describe tumors originating from this type of cell.

Brain tumors can often be identified more specifically, and once they are can then be given a name describing the exact type of cell the tumor originated from. Gliomas, for example, can originate from any of the supporting cells, so a glioma may be further classified as an astrocytoma (originating from astrocytes), oligodendroglioma (originating from oligodendroctyes), and so on. Thus, the group of brain tumors known as gliomas contains many different subtypes of tumors, each identified by exactly which type of glial cell it arose from.

Classifying the tumor by its cell of origin is important because knowing the type of cell giving rise to the tumor allows doctors to predict how the tumor will behave to some degree. There are several different classification systems in use, but the one most commonly used is that developed by the World Health Organization (Table 10.1).

TUMOR GRADE

Even tumors originating from the same type of cell will behave differently. For example, some astrocytomas are completely benign while others grow rapidly and spread throughout the brain in a matter of months. How rapidly a certain tumor is expected to grow and spread is referred to as the degree of malignancy or the tumor's grade. The grade of an individual tumor can be determined only by examining cells from the tumor under a microscope. By observing whether certain characteristics are present in the tumor cells, a pathologist can decide what grade the tumor is.

Each category of tumor (astrocytoma, meningioma, etc.) has its own grading criteria, but for all tumor types the grade is represented by a Roman numeral from I to III or I to IV. Lower grade tumors appear similar to normal cells, tend to grow more slowly, and are less likely to spread into surrounding tissue. Higher grade tumors appear quite different from normal cells, grow very quickly, and are likely to spread into surrounding tissues. Middle grade tumors fall somewhere between these two.

Tumors often contain several different grades of cells. The highest or most malignant grade of cell found during microscopic

Table 10.1   Categories of Central Nervous System Tumors by the Cells of Origin*

1 Tumors of Glial Cell Origin
   1.1 Astrocytic tumors (astrocytoma, glioblastoma)
   1.2 Oligodendroglial tumors (oligodendroglioma)
   1.3 Ependymal tumors (ependymoma)
   1.4 Mixed Gliomas (oligo-astrocytoma)
   1.5 Choroid plexus tumors
   1.6 Neuroepithelial tumors of uncertain origin
   1.7 Neuronal and mixed neuronal-glial tumors (gangliocytoma, ganglioglioma)
   1.8 Pineal parenchymal tumors (pineocytoma, pineoblastoma)
   1.9 Embryonal tumors (neuroblastoma, medulloblastoma)

2 Tumors of Cranial and Spinal Nerves (Neurofibroma, Malignant Schwannoma)

3 Tumors of the Meninges
   3.1 Tumors of the meningothelial cells (meningioma, malignant meningioma)
   3.2 Mesenchymal, nonmeningothelial tumors
   3.3 Benign neoplasms (lipoma, fibrous histiocytoma)
   3.4 Malignant neoplasms (hemangiopericytoma, malignant fibrous histiocytoma)
   3.5 Primary melanocytic lesions
   3.6 Tumors of uncertain (hemangioblastoma)

4 Lymphomas and Hemopoietic Neoplasms

5 Germ Cell Tumors (Choriocarcinoma, Teratoma, Mixed Germ Cell Tumors)

6 Cysts and Tumorlike Lesions (Epidermoid cyst, Dermoid cyst)

7 Tumors of the Sellar Region
   7.1 Pituitary adenoma
   7.2 Pituitary carcinoma
   7.3 Craniopharyngioma

8 Local Extensions from Regional Tumors

9 Metastatic Tumors

10 Unclassified Tumors

This table doesn't demonstrate all the dozens of subcategories of the actual WHO classification, but it covers all the more common primary brain tumor types.

examination decides the tumors overall grade, even if most of the tumor cells are a lower grade. This is because over time the highest grade (and therefore most rapidly growing) cells will become the most common type of cell in the tumor.

Specific Types of Primary Brain Tumors

About half of all brain tumors are secondary tumors. The treatment and outcome of these tumors depends upon the type of cancer they have originated from and whether that cancer has spread to other parts of the body. Generally, if the brain appears to be the only area of metastasis, the tumor will be treated with surgery (see chapter 12) and any other treatments that the primary tumor is known to respond to.

The most common types of primary brain tumors are those originating from the glial cells—the supporting cells of the brain. These tumors include astrocytoma, medulloblastoma, ependymoma, and others (see Table 10.1 on page 149). Together, glial cell tumors account for about 60 percent of all adult brain tumors. Tumors arising from the meninges (the covering membranes of the brain) account for just under 20 percent of all adult brain tumors, making them the second most common category of primary brain tumors in adults. The third most common type of adult brain tumors are pituitary tumors, which account for about 15 percent of primary brain tumors.

The types of brain tumors that occur in children are different from those that occur in adults. Children are about as likely as adults to have tumors originating from the glial cells, but childhood tumors are more likely to be primitive and malignant tumors called neuroblastoma and medulloblastoma. Children are less likely to have pituitary and meningeal tumors than adults, and more likely to have germ-cell tumors (congenital tumors caused by abnormalities during development) and cystic (hollow) tumors (see Table 10.1).

Tumors of the Glial Cells

Glial cell tumors often originate in the cerebral hemispheres, particularly in the frontal and parietal lobes, but can occur anywhere in the brain. Tumors originating from astrocyte cells (see chapter 1) are by far the most common subtype of glial cell tumors, accounting for more than 80 percent of all gliomas.

ASTROCYTOMA AND GLIOBLASTOMA

Astrocytomas and glioblastomas are tumors that arise from astrocytes, the cells that provide the brain's connective tissue structure. The grading of these tumors for degree of malignancy is somewhat confusing because several different systems are in use. The more commonly used system, the World Health organization classification, separates these tumors into three grades:

1. Well-differentiated astrocytomas
2. Anaplastic (meaning poorly differentiated) astrocytomas
3. Glioblastoma (also called glioblastoma multiforme)

The older grading systems use four grades:

1. Benign pilocytic astrocytoma
2. Well-differentiated astrocytoma
3. Anaplastic astrocytoma
4. Glioblastoma

With either system, lower-grade tumors are less malignant. Occasionally, astrocytomas are mixed with other types of cancerous glial cells. These types of tumors are referred to as mixed gliomas.

Well-Differentiated Astrocytoma
These astrocytomas usually have well-defined borders or are enclosed in a cyst (a hollow, fluid-filled ball). The two lowest-grade

astrocytomas are sometimes called juvenile pilocytic astrocytomas and subependymal giant cell astrocytomas. Juvenile pilocytic astrocytomas occur mainly in children, often beginning in the cerebellum or near the optic nerve. They often have a cyst-like appearance. Unless their location prevents removal, these tumors are benign.

Infiltrating well-differentiated astrocytomas, also referred to as low-grade astrocytomas, are more malignant. They are often found in the temporal lobe of the cerebral hemispheres, but may occur in any part of the brain.

Complete surgical removal of a well-differentiated astrocytoma is sometimes possible, and in these cases the tumor rarely recurs. Some of these tumors are located in areas of the brain that prevent their removal without causing severe neurological damage, however. Radiation therapy is used for incompletely removed or inoperable low-grade astrocytomas, and for those that recur after surgical removal. The average length of survival after diagnosis of a well-differentiated astrocytoma is about five years. Happily, many patients with this type of tumor are completely cured.

CASE STUDY: Astrocytoma

Bill had noticed a bit of weakness in his left arm for a month or so, but hadn't really considered it a problem. He had also complained of generally feeling bad, but really had no particular symptoms. He thought that perhaps he was overtired from work. Without any other warning, Bill suddenly had a seizure at work, completely collapsing and having generalized convulsions. One of his coworkers called an ambulance, and Bill was taken to the hospital.

An MRI scan showed that Bill had a tumor in the right side of his brain. Because of the tumor's appearance on the MRI scan, doctors suspected it was malignant. They recommended a craniotomy and surgical removal of the tumor, with a frozen section (a biopsy performed and examined during the surgery). The frozen section was examined by a pathologist who determined the tumor was an infiltrating astrocytoma, a low-grade malignant tumor. The surgeon was able to remove all the visible tumor.

Following surgery, Bill had even more weakness in his left arm. He began physical therapy, and within a few weeks most of the function of his arm had returned. His neurosurgeon recommended that Bill undergo radiation therapy to destroy any remaining tumor cells. He has had about half of his radiation treatments and, other than a bit of nausea, has experienced no problems.

The neurosurgeon has told Bill there is about a 50 percent chance that the tumor will never come back. He will undergo a repeat MRI scan in six months and again at one year and every year afterwards. If the tumor does return, Bill may require further surgery or radiation, or it may be treated with chemotherapy. Although the tumor will probably be lethal if it does return, chances are that Bill will survive at least five years, even if the tumor recurs.

Poorly Differentiated Astrocytoma

Poorly differentiated astrocytomas (also called gemistocytic astrocytoma, anaplastic astrocytoma, and malignant astrocytoma) are truly malignant tumors. They grow more rapidly than well-differentiated tumors and frequently invade nearby healthy tissue. They are more likely to recur because their tendency to spread into surrounding tissues makes it difficult to remove them completely during surgery.

Treatment is based upon the amount the tumor has spread when the diagnosis is made. Surgery followed by radiation therapy is the most common treatment for high-grade astrocytomas. If the location of the tumor mitigates against surgery, high-dose radiation therapy is administered. Chemotherapy may be used in addition to surgery and/or radiation therapy. Investigational immunotherapy treatments are also available.

The combination of surgery, radiation, and chemotherapy has become quite effective in treating these tumors. Over 80 percent of patients with poorly differentiated astrocytoma will survive more than one year, and about 40 percent will live three years or more.

Glioblastoma

The highest grade of astrocyte tumor is the glioblastoma (also called glioblastoma multiforme), one of the most malignant and difficult brain tumors to treat. This is a poorly differentiated (meaning it doesn't resemble astrocytes), rapidly growing, and highly invasive tumor. Glioblastoma is the most common primary brain tumor found in middle-aged adults, causing 30 percent of all primary brain tumors in this age group.

Surgery alone cannot remove a glioblastoma because the tumor cells rapidly invade tissues throughout the brain. Surgery may be performed to debulk the tumor, however. Debulking surgery removes as much of the tumor as can be easily reached without attempting to remove it all. While debulking cannot cure the cancer, it prolongs life expectancy and improves quality of life in most cases. After debulking, whole brain radiation is administered, often followed by chemotherapy.

Unfortunately, each glioblastoma contains a mixture of several different cell types, which makes it particularly difficult to treat. While one cell type may respond to a certain treatment and die, other cell types will be unaffected by that particular treatment. The one-year survival rate for patients with glioblastoma is about 60 percent, but the five-year survival rate is less than 20 percent. A variation of glioblastoma, the gliosarcoma, behaves similarly.

Location of Astrocytic Tumors

The location of a glial tumor within the brain can be an important factor in predicting its outcome. The most common location for astrocytic tumors is in the cerebral hemispheres, but they are sometimes found in the cerebellum. In general, cerebellar tumors are more curable than those originating in the cerebral hemispheres.

Any glial tumor located in the brain stem (it may be a well-differentiated or poorly differentiated astrocytoma, or glioblastoma) is generally referred to as a brain stem glioma, because in this case the location is more important than the tumor type. Brain stem gliomas are usually diagnosed simply by evidence from MRI scans because biopsy might be hazardous. They are more common in children than in adults.

Because of their location, brain stem tumors are almost always inoperable. The treatment of choice is radiation therapy, although chemotherapy may also be attempted.

Astrocytomas sometimes occur in the optic nerve (the nerve that carries vision messages from eyeball to brain), usually in children under the age of ten. The tumors are usually benign when they occur in this area, but occasionally are malignant. When the tumor involves only one optic nerve, surgery is the treatment of choice, but it will result in blindness of the affected eye. Given that surgery will result in complete blindness, radiation therapy is the treatment of choice if the tumor is located at the junction of the two optic nerves. Chemotherapy may also be given.

OLIGODENDROGLIOMA

These tumors arise from the oligodendrocytes, the supporting cells of the brain that form the covering of axons and dendrites. Oligodendrogliomas are not as common as astrocytomas, but still account for 4 percent of all primary brain tumors. They tend to occur in middle-aged individuals and are usually located in one of the cerebral hemispheres.

Pure oligodendrogliomas are usually slow-growing, low-grade tumors that are often present for many years before they are detected. They can occasionally be a high-grade malignancy, however. The treatment of choice is surgical removal of as much of the tumor as possible, followed by radiation therapy. Chemotherapy remains under investigation but at this point does not appear very effective. Recurrence of the tumor is not unusual, but because it grows so slowly the average patient survives four to five years after the diagnosis is made. A complete cure is possible if the tumor can be removed completely by surgery.

EPENDYMAL TUMORS

Ependymal tumors originate from the ependymal cells that line the ventricles in the brain. About 5 percent of all intracranial tumors are ependymomas. They usually occur during childhood or adolescence.

Ependymomas vary in their grade of malignancy. Most are benign or low-grade malignancies that are often curable by surgical removal. Anaplastic ependymoma is a more malignant type of ependymoma. The most malignant form of ependymal tumor is ependymoblastoma, a rare tumor of childhood that grows very rapidly and is difficult to treat.

Treatment for low-grade ependymoma is surgical resection followed by radiation. Some evidence suggests that patients with anaplastic ependymoma who are treated with both surgery and radiation do nearly as well as patients with low-grade ependymomas. Chemotherapy is used to treat recurring tumors, and new clinical trials are using chemotherapy for initial treatment along with surgery and radiation.

Because ependymomas are located inside the ventricles, they may block the flow of cerebrospinal fluid, causing hydrocephalus (water on the brain). In these cases, surgeons may need to place a shunt—an internal tube to drain fluid—past the obstruction.

MIXED GLIOMA

Mixed gliomas are tumors containing more than one type of cell. The most common mixed gliomas contain either astrocytes and oligodendrocytes, or astrocytes and ependymoma cells. Mixed gliomas are treated according to the highest grade of cells found in the tumor. In general, the highest grade of cells will be poorly differentiated astrocytoma cells. Mixed gliomas may have similar outcomes to those tumors.

CHOROID PLEXUS TUMORS

The choroid plexus is an area inside the ventricles of the brain that produces cerebrospinal fluid. Tumors of the choroid plexus occur primarily in very young children, particularly those under age two. There are two types of choroid plexus tumors: choroid plexus papilloma is a slow-growing benign tumor; choroid plexus carcinoma is a fast-growing, malignant tumor.

The first sign of a choroid plexus tumor is hydrocephalus due to obstruction of cerebrospinal fluid flow, which occurs early. Since choroid plexus tumors usually occur in very young children who cannot express their symptoms very well, the first signs are usually irritability, inability to focus the eyes, and altered consciousness. Complete surgical removal of a choroid plexus papilloma almost always results in complete cure. Carcinomas require surgery, radiation, and chemotherapy. The majority of carcinomas are cured, but a cure is less likely if they have spread to other areas of the brain.

GANGLIOGLIOMAS

Gangliogliomas are slow-growing tumors that frequently occur in the temporal lobe, although they can be found anywhere in the brain. They are most likely to develop in older children and adolescents. Because they are slow growing, many children suffer seizures for several years before the tumor is finally diagnosed. Intellectual and behavioral difficulties may also occur, especially in temporal lobe gangliogliomas. Surgical removal of the tumor is usually curative, but radiation may also be used in some treatment centers.

Tumors of the Meningeal Membranes

Tumors of the meningeal membranes, the connective tissue coverings of the brain, comprise the second most common type of primary brain tumor. The majority are benign and can be removed completely by surgery. Other meningeal tumors consist of benign cells but cannot be removed completely because of their location. Only 5 to 10 percent of meningeal tumors are malignant and spread to other areas of the brain.

MENINGIOMA

These tumors arise from cells in the meningeal membranes that cover the brain. Meningiomas are slow-growing tumors that can become quite large before symptoms appear. Benign meningiomas can compress normal brain tissue and do not invade the brain itself. If they become large enough, however, they can erode the bones of the skull. Malignant meningiomas, although rare, do invade brain tissue.

The symptoms produced by meningiomas depend on their size, location, and growth rate. Rapidly growing tumors are more likely to cause symptoms early in their course, while slow-growing tumors often become large before causing significant symptoms.

Meningiomas can usually be removed completely by surgery, but in some cases the tumor's location makes removal impossible without damaging vital structures. When the tumor is removed, the chance of it recurring is less than 10 percent. When it cannot be removed completely, radiation therapy is used to slow its growth. Recent research suggests that new types of chemotherapy based on drugs interfering with the hormone progesterone can also slow the growth of these tumors. Even when removal is incomplete, more than 50 percent of meningioma patients remain alive ten years after the original diagnosis.

CASE STUDY: Meningioma

John, a forty-seven-year-old businessman, noticed that his golf game was deteriorating because he couldn't grip his clubs well. Over the next year, he found that his left hand became increasingly weak. A few times he dropped things, and he had difficulty using his computer because of problems typing with his left hand. He saw his doctor, who took x-rays of his wrist that were normal. The doctor ordered a nerve conduction test to check for carpal tunnel syndrome (a nerve entrapment of the hand that can occur in people who type a lot). The test was normal, and the doctor recommended that John have physical therapy for tendinitis in his hand and forearm. He also started him on arthritis medicine.

A month after finishing therapy, John noticed he was having headaches on the right side of his head. Because he was under a lot of pressure at work, he decided the headaches were stress-related. A few weeks later he began feeling nauseous in the morning and noticed he had double vision when working late one night. He saw his doctor again who ordered a CT scan of John's head. The scan showed a large meningioma on the right side of the brain. John underwent a craniotomy and the tumor was completely removed. Microscopic examination of the tumor indicated that it was benign, and no other treatment was necessary.

John's headaches and double vision cleared up completely within a few days after surgery, and his left hand and arm slowly regained strength over several months. They were still a bit weaker than his right, but much improved compared to the year before surgery. John had a repeat CT scan a year after surgery and no tumor was seen.

HEMANGIOBLASTOMA

Hemangioblastoma is a benign tumor arising from the cells lining the brain's blood vessels. It is a rare tumor, accounting for only about

2 percent of all primary brain tumors and occurring most frequently in persons thirty-five to forty-five years old. The most common site of hemangioblastoma is the cerebellum. It is slow growing and does not metastasize.

Surgical removal is the treatment of choice for this tumor. Angiography (see chapter 4) is done before surgery to confirm diagnosis and provide information about the tumor's blood supply. If the tumor cannot be removed completely because of its location, it can be treated effectively with radiation therapy.

Tumors of the Pituitary Gland

The pituitary gland hangs beneath the center of the brain (see Fig. 1.4 on page 13). The gland is really two separate organs combined in one location. The posterior lobe of the gland is connected directly to the brain and controls hormones that regulate the body's water balance. The front half consists of a different type of tissue. This lobe secretes chemicals that control levels of many different hormones in the body including estrogen, progesterone, growth hormone, steroids, and thyroid hormone.

Tumors of the pituitary are adenomas (tumors arising from glandular tissue). Pituitary adenomas cause 8 percent of all primary brain tumors and are most common in young or middle-aged adults. Almost all these tumors are benign and very slow growing, although on occasion they can prove to be malignant.

Pituitary adenomas are classified according to their cell of origin as are other brain tumors. Unlike them, pituitary adenomas are further classified as secreting or nonsecreting, depending upon whether they release the hormone made by their cell of origin. The majority of pituitary adenomas are secreting tumors.

Secreting tumors usually cause early symptoms because of the hormones they release (see Table 10.2). The most common type of pi-

Table 10.2   Hormonal Problems Caused by Pituitary Tumors

Acromegaly   Caused by pituitary tumors that secrete growth hormone
  if they occur after puberty. Bones in the hands, feet, and jaws become
  enlarged.

Gigantism   Caused by pituitary tumors that secrete growth hormone if
  they occur before puberty. People become extremely tall, often with
  large hands, protruding jaw and eyebrows, and severe arthritis.

Cushing's disease   Caused by tumors secreting ACTH (Adrenal Corti-
  cotrophin Hormone). Patients develop a moon-shaped face and fat deposits on the back of the neck, stretch marks in the skin, pimples, and
  high blood pressure.

Prolactin syndrome   Caused by pituitary tumors secreting prolactin,
  the most common type of pituitary tumor. Production of breast milk in
  women who are not pregnant, loss of menstrual cycle, and loss of
  bone calcium are all hallmarks of this tumor. Many women with this
  tumor visit their gynecologist thinking that they might be pregnant.

Growth hormone secreting tumors   May very occasionally be treated
  with drugs but most often must be removed surgically.

tuitary adenoma secretes prolactin. This tumor will usually cause impotence in males while females will experience loss of their menstrual
periods and secretion of breast milk. The second most common pituitary adenoma secretes growth hormone, which causes enlargement of
the hands, feet, and jaw. In some people, excess growth hormone can
also cause symptoms similar to diabetes. Less common types of pituitary tumors can cause secretion of excessive amounts of cortisone or
thyroid hormone.

Nonsecreting adenomas usually don't cause symptoms until they
are large enough to put pressure on the optic nerves, which pass just
above the pituitary gland. The most common symptoms in people
with these tumors are loss of vision and headache.

Almost all pituitary tumors have a good outcome, but treatment of the tumors varies depending upon their type. Prolactin-secreting adenomas usually respond to medications that stop the symptoms and shrink the tumor. When medication works successfully, no other treatment is required. Other types of secreting pituitary tumors are treated by surgical removal. Unlike most brain tumors, removal of pituitary tumors does not require a craniotomy.

When surgery cannot be performed because of a patient's overall condition, secreting pituitary tumors can be treated by radiation, especially given the newer forms of radiation therapy available. Unfortunately, radiation therapy may cause loss of function in the remainder of the pituitary gland requiring patients to depend on hormone supplements. Radiation is also not likely to correct vision losses in patients with large tumors.

Nonsecreting tumors are likely to be quite large by the time they are diagnosed. Surgical removal is the treatment of choice and results in a complete cure in most cases. If the tumor is very large, partial surgical removal followed by radiation therapy usually proves effective.

Other Brain Tumors

CRANIOPHARYNGIOMAS

Craniopharyngioma is a tumor that arises from the remains of a structure found in the developing embryo. Although they occur in the region of the pituitary gland, they do not behave like pituitary tumors. The tumor causes symptoms by pressing on the optic nerves, resulting in loss of vision. It may also obstruct cerebrospinal fluid flow, causing hydrocephalus.

Craniopharyngiomas are always benign and are most common in children and adolescents. They are localized tumors that grow slowly and never metastasize, although they can erode into nearby structures. Surgical removal is the treatment of choice but may not be possible in some cases because of the tumor's location. Radiation therapy is used only if the tumor cannot be removed completely by surgery.

TUMORS OF THE PINEAL GLAND

The pineal gland is located above and behind the thalamus in the center of the brain. Pineal tumors are rare in adults, causing less than 1 percent of all primary brain tumors. They are more common in children, however, causing 3 to 8 percent of childhood brain tumors. For unknown reasons, tumors in this region tend to consist of cells normally seen only in a developing fetus, which are known as embryonal cells.

The most common pineal tumor is the germinoma, which accounts for about 30 percent of the tumors in this region. They are most common in teenagers. Other pineal tumors include teratomas, astrocytomas, pineocytomas, and pineoblastomas.

Because of their location, pineal tumors are likely to obstruct the flow of cerebrospinal fluid, causing hydrocephalus. Symptoms include headache, nausea and vomiting, and double vision. Pineal tumors are also unique in that they can be diagnosed by analyzing for certain chemical markers in the spinal fluid.

Surgery is occasionally used to completely remove pineal tumors, but usually only a small piece of the tumor is removed—a biopsy—to determine the specific type of tumor. Most pineal tumors respond very well to radiation therapy, especially germinomas. If hydrocephalus is present, a shunt procedure (see chapter 12) to allow cerebrospinal fluid to drain may also be necessary. Chemotherapy for pineoblastomas and germinomas is presently under investigation.

MEDULLOBLASTOMA

Medulloblastoma arises from one of the cells of the developing brain—cells that normally disappear before birth. Because it arises

from this cell type it is classified as one of the primitive neuroecto-
derm (the fetal tissue that gives rise to the brain) tumors. Medulloblastoma is probably the second most common type of brain tumor
affecting children, accounting for 20 percent of all pediatric brain tumors. It most commonly occurs between ages four and eight, but can
occur in any age group, including adults. It is twice as common in
males as in females.

Medulloblastoma grows rapidly and is quite malignant, metastasizing to other parts of the brain through the cerebrospinal fluid. The
tumor may actually metastasize out of the brain into other parts of the
body, one of the few primary brain tumors known to do so.

Medulloblastomas almost always start in the middle of the cerebellum (see Fig. 1.2 or 1.4 on pages 9 and 13). Tumors in this location
are likely to block cerebrospinal fluid flow and cause symptoms of hydrocephalus such as double vision, headaches, and nausea. In small
children medulloblastoma may cause the eyes to become fixed in a
downward gaze because the tumor often presses on a brain location
that affects visual control.

Treatment of medulloblastoma depends upon the tumor's stage—
a system that measures how large the tumor has grown and how far it
has spread. Treatment always includes surgical removal of as much of
the tumor as possible. Radiation of the tumor area as well as the entire brain and spinal cord follows, given that the tumor is very sensitive to radiation. Chemotherapy may also be used, particularly in very
young children. Surgery and radiation treatment is repeated whenever the tumor recurs. It is often necessary to place a shunt, since this
tumor often causes hydrocephalus.

ACOUSTIC NEUROMA

Acoustic neuroma is a benign tumor involving the nerve of hearing
(known as the acoustic nerve, or eighth cranial nerve). This nerve enters the brain in the angle between the cerebellum and the pons (see

Fig. 1.3 on page 11). They account for about 9 percent of all brain tumors and usually occur in middle-aged adults. It is twice as common in females as in males.

Acoustic neuroma grows very slowly so its symptoms tend to be minor at first. Over time, affected persons experience buzzing or ringing in the ear, followed by loss of hearing in one ear. Some people also experience dizziness, facial numbness or weakness, and some have headaches on the affected side of their head. Treatment of acoustic neuroma is usually total surgical removal, which completely cures the tumor. In some cases, focused beam radiation therapy (see chapter 13) can be used instead of surgery.

Because this tumor grows within the acoustic nerve, permanent deafness in the affected ear may result from either surgery or radiation. Weakness of facial muscles may also occur following treatment but usually recovers over time.

DERMOID AND EPIDERMOID CYSTS

Dermoid cysts are more common in the spinal cord than the brain. Dermoid cysts in the brain are most likely to occur in children under age ten, while those in the spine are most likely to occur between ages ten and twenty. Dermoid cysts are almost always benign and can (generally) be removed completely by surgery. If they return, they grow very slowly.

Epidermoid cysts are more common than dermoid cysts and are usually found in the brain rather than in the spine. They most commonly occur in middle-aged adults. They are generally benign and are surgically removed if possible.

CENTRAL NERVOUS SYSTEM LYMPHOMA

Lymphoma is actually a solid tumor of the white blood cells. When it occurs in the brain, lymphoma most often begins in one of the cerebral hemispheres. In some cases, the tumor is found in more than one location within the brain, and metastasis may occur anywhere in the brain. Symptoms include confusion, lethargy, memory loss, and often muscle weakness in one area of the body.

Lymphoma is particularly common in people whose immune system is not functioning properly. This includes people who have had organ transplants and those with AIDS, among others. For unknown reasons, the incidence of central nervous system lymphoma is increasing, even in people with healthy immune systems.

Surgical removal of the tumor may be required to remove pressure in the affected area of the brain, or to obtain tissue for a biopsy. Surgery is not curative, however. These tumors are sensitive to radiation therapy, and steroids and chemotherapy may also be used. Unfortunately, the blood–brain barrier may prevent standard chemotherapy from actually reaching the tumor. Several methods of administering chemotherapy that allow medications to cross the blood–brain barrier are being developed, however.

CHORDOMA

Chordoma is a rare tumor that occurs only at the base of the skull. Although it is benign, it frequently invades the adjacent bones of the skull. It most often occurs in people ages twenty-one to forty. A complete surgical resection is often possible for this tumor, with radiation therapy usually administered following surgery.

Secondary (Metastatic) Brain Tumors

Tumors from other parts of the body often spread to the brain. In fact, metastatic (or secondary) brain tumors are slightly more common than all primary brain tumors combined. The most common causes of metastatic brain tumors are cancers of the lung, breast, kidney, and skin. In some cases, the symptoms caused by metastatic brain tumor are the first sign that a primary tumor exists.

Most tumors spread to the brain through the bloodstream. Once they begin to grow within the brain, they cause swelling of the brain tissue. The exact symptoms will depend upon the location of the tumor. Hydrocephalus and increased intracranial pressure symptoms (headache, irritability, nausea) occur if the tumor is located near one of the ventricles. Seizures or stroke-like symptoms may occur if the tumor is in the cerebral cortex.

Usually a single metastatic tumor is found in the brain, although there may be multiple metastatic tumors. A single metastasis is usually removed by surgery, especially if the primary tumor is curable. If there are multiple metastatic tumors, or if the primary tumor is not curable, radiation therapy is employed.

CHAPTER 11

The Symptoms and Diagnosis of Brain Tumors

The Symptoms of Brain Tumors

Brain tumors are difficult to diagnose for several reasons. Obviously, since they are located inside the skull, there is no lump or mass that a doctor can feel or that leads to a suspicion that there might be a tumor. Symptoms are often vague and usually start very slowly. Many people ignore them for a long time in the belief that they will just go away. Additionally, the symptoms produced by a brain tumor often mimic those of other diseases. Since brain tumors are not very common, your doctor will often investigate other (likely) causes before considering a brain tumor as a possibility.

In general, the symptoms of a brain tumor depend on its size and the region of the brain in which it is located. As the tumor grows, it presses on brain structures, causing them to function abnormally and slowly producing more and more symptoms. Because the symptoms appear gradually, and it is usually not clear that they are caused by a brain tumor, it may be a long time between the onset of symptoms and an accurate diagnosis.

There are exceptions, however. The blood vessels to the tumor, which are thin-walled and weak, may burst, causing the sudden symptoms of a hemorrhagic stroke. Sometimes the tumor obstructs the flow of cerebrospinal fluid, which rapidly causes the symptoms of increased intracranial pressure. Certain specific tumor types, particularly those of the pituitary gland, secrete abnormal hormones or other substances that cause significant symptoms before the tumor is actually large enough to interfere with brain function.

THE MASS EFFECT

Most symptoms caused by brain tumors are due to the tumor's size. Because the skull is made of hard bone, it cannot expand to accommodate a growing tumor. Therefore, a brain tumor will always press on some part of the brain. As the tumor grows, it compresses normal brain tissue causing it to function abnormally, or stop functioning altogether.

Depending upon the tumor's location, the mass effect may cause very specific symptoms when the tumor is still quite small, or may cause few symptoms even if the tumor is large. For example, a tumor one centimeter (about ⅓ inch) in diameter located in the brain stem will almost always cause significant symptoms. On the other hand, a meningioma (tumor of the brain's covering tissue) located over the frontal lobes may grow to be several inches in diameter while causing only vague symptoms such as headache or forgetfulness.

In some cases, the tumor will cause some sudden change within the brain that immediately increases the symptoms of the mass effect. The most common events that can result in a sudden change are:

- Bleeding into the tumor
- Swelling within the tumor

• Blockage of the flow of cerebrospinal fluid

Bleeding into the tumor is common only in fairly large tumors, or in those that have a very rich blood supply. When such bleeding occurs, the signs and symptoms are similar to that of a hemorrhagic stroke. The person's level of consciousness may suddenly decrease, they may experience nausea and vomiting, or they may have a sudden headache.

Tumors that grow rapidly may outgrow their own blood supply, causing many of the tumor cells to die. Whenever a large number of tumor cells die, a large amount of swelling occurs, similar to the swelling effect in normal brain tissue after a stroke. Swelling can also result when the tumor cells invade normal brain tissue and cause that area to become irritated. In either case, swelling increases the mass effect, thus causing more symptoms to develop.

Whether the mass effect develops quickly or slowly, it produces two types of symptoms. The first are the generalized symptoms of increased intracranial pressure (pressure within the skull). The second type develop specifically in the area nearest the tumor. In some cases the specific symptoms are much more pronounced than the generalized symptoms; in others almost no specific symptoms develop.

General Symptoms of Increased Intracranial Pressure

Tumors in certain locations can block the flow of cerebrospinal fluid around and through the brain. When this occurs, fluid "backs up" behind the blockage, causing hydrocephalus, which increases pressure within the skull. If the blockage occurs over a short period of time, such as would occur if a tumor bleeds into itself or swells suddenly, the symptoms of hydrocephalus quickly become severe. If the blockage occurs slowly, as a tumor grows steadily and slowly obstructs the flow of fluid, the brain will compensate for the increased pressure to some degree. In this circumstance the symptoms of hydrocephalus will be less dramatic.

There are several common symptoms of increased intracranial pressure. Headache is perhaps the most common symptom, with the headache usually worse in the morning and lessening in intensity during the day. Nausea and vomiting may also occur, and again, the symptom is usually worse early in the morning. As the pressure increases, mental changes including drowsiness, sluggish thinking, and loss of coordination may become apparent. Double vision is another symptom, but it is usually a late sign that occurs only after the pressure has become quite high.

Specific Mass Effect in Certain Locations

Brain Stem Tumors   Tumors of the brain stem are very likely to cause the symptoms of increased intracranial pressure since they will almost always obstruct the flow of cerebrospinal fluid. Persons with tumors in the brain stem often develop a clumsy, uncoordinated gait or muscle weakness on one side of the body. Tumors in the upper brain stem and pons can cause muscle weakness on one side of the face, difficulty with swallowing and/or speaking, and episodes of crossed eyes with double vision.

Cerebral Hemisphere Tumors   Tumors of the cerebral hemisphere can cause a wide range of symptoms depending upon which lobe of the hemisphere they affect. Cerebral hemisphere tumors, in general, are not as likely to cause signs of increased intracranial pressure as are tumors in other locations. Tumors of the cerebral hemispheres are more likely to cause seizures than tumors in other locations, however. The seizures may be generalized grand mal seizures (the entire body is involved), or they may be focal seizures that involve only one extremity or one part of the body. Seizures are the first symptom of tumor in the cerebral hemisphere in 20 percent of cases. In any person over age forty who develops seizures, a complete evaluation for brain tumor should be performed.

Tumors involving the frontal lobes may cause weakness in one part of the body, which can progress to complete paralysis over time. Memory lapses, impaired judgment, and personality or emotional changes may also occur. These changes often develop slowly over several months and may be attributed—initially—to aging or stress. If the tumor is located underneath the frontal lobe, loss of the sense of smell or a change of vision may also occur.

Parietal lobe tumors are particularly likely to cause seizures. If the tumor is in the dominant hemisphere, problems with understanding speech, writing, or reading may develop. Tumors in the nondominant parietal lobe may cause problems recognizing the orientation of objects in space (angles and distance), or even an inability to recognize body parts.

Occipital lobe tumors are also likely to cause seizures and sometimes result in blindness in one direction. (Blindness in one direction means that both eyes cannot see to one side.) Temporal lobe tumors often cause no symptoms other than seizures or problems with speech. Some temporal lobe tumors cause unexpected fits of emotion or temporal lobe epilepsy, periods of bizarre or unusual behavior that the person cannot remember.

If the tumor originates in the deeper parts of the cerebral cortex, it will generally cause paralysis and loss of sensation to one side of the body. Additionally, these tumors are more likely to cause the symptoms of increased intracranial pressure compared to other tumors of the cerebral cortex.

Midline Tumors (Craniopharyngioma, Thalamic Tumors, Pituitary Tumors)   These tumors are likely to cause vision changes because the optic chiasm, the location where the two optic nerves cross each other (see Fig. 1.4 on page 13), is located in this area. Loss of peripheral vision is a common symptom. These tumors are also likely to cause the generalized symptoms of increased intracranial pressure including headaches and nausea. Other symptoms include abnormal eye movements and changes in personality in a few cases. The development of diabetes insipidus (inability of the body to regulate its water supply) may also occur, as can other hormonal problems (see below).

Cerebellar Tumors   Cerebellar tumors are sometimes referred to as posterior fossa tumors because the cerebellum resides in a separate compartment (or fossa) in the back of the head. Tumors in this location are very likely to cause the symptoms associated with increased intracranial pressure. A clumsy, uncoordinated walk or even staggering may also occur. Coordination of the arms may also be impaired, and speech may be slurred. A specific type of tremor that occurs only when an extremity is being moved, such as when reaching for an object, called an intention tremor, may also be present. In addition to the type of headache that accompanies increased intracranial pressure, there may be a deep aching pain at the base of the skull or top of the neck.

Acoustic Nerve Tumors   The earliest symptom of acoustic neuroma is usually a ringing or buzzing in the ear. Occasionally, dizziness (vertigo) or loss of hearing in one ear may occur. When the tumor grows larger, it may cause all the symptoms present in brain-stem tumors.

CHANGE IN HORMONE FUNCTION

Everyone is aware that certain glands in our body produce hormones that help regulate various functions. The thyroid gland produces hormones that regulate metabolism, for example, and the ovary secretes estrogen and progesterone regulating a woman's monthly cycle (Table 11.1). The amount of hormone that a gland produces is regulated by chemicals called releasing factors circulating in the bloodstream. These chemicals are produced and released by the pituitary gland at the base of the brain. The pituitary also directly produces some hormones such as growth hormone, and the various hormones that regulate fluid and salt balance within the body.

Table 11.1   Some Hormones Produced by the Pituitary Gland

Hormone Name	Function
Growth Hormone (GH)	Stimulates growth of body tissues Raises blood sugar levels Increases some types of body metabolism
Adrenocorticotrophic	Causes the adrenal gland to release cortisones
ACTH Hormone	Controls metabolism and fluid balance
Thyrotrophic Hormone (TH)	Causes the thyroid gland to release hormones that increase metabolism
Prolactin	Stimulates breasts to produce milk
Melanocyte-Stimulating Hormone	Controls the skin's pigment
Antidiuretic Hormone (ADH)	Reduces the amount of urine

Tumors involving the pituitary gland often cause symptoms affecting the entire body because they either release hormones abnormally or prevent hormones from being released properly. These tumors can produce a variety of different problems. If the tumor itself secretes a hormone or releasing factor, symptoms of hormone excess may appear soon after the tumor begins. If it does not secrete hormones, it may eventually destroy the other cells in the pituitary gland, causing the symptoms resulting from a lack of hormones.

Growth Disorders

Growth disorders will obviously be more apparent in children, although they can also affect adults to some degree. Short stature is a common presenting symptom of children who have tumors that damage the pituitary's ability to secrete growth hormone. Failure to grow may also occur in children who have received radiation or undergone surgery for tumors in the area of the pituitary gland. Treatment with growth hormone can restore growth for most children with growth hormone deficiency.

Rare pituitary tumors that secrete growth hormone cause excessive growth. If not treated these tumors result in gigantism. Because some bones are more sensitive to this hormone than others, the body's overall growth is usually not proportional. The person affected has very large hands and feet, a large jaw, and jutting eyebrows.

Acromegaly occurs when too much growth hormone is secreted in an adult. Since the long bones of the body are no longer capable of growth, enlargement only occurs in the hands, feet, and jaw. The tongue often becomes thicker and may interfere with speech. Acromegaly can also cause high blood pressure and heart disease if not treated.

Disorders of Sexual Development

If a pituitary tumor causes the release of excess sexual hormones, puberty may begin even in very young children, a condition called precocious puberty. The affected child will develop all the secondary sex characteristics of their gender (body hair, breast development, menstruation, etc.). If the process is not stopped (medication is effective until primary treatment of the tumor can be started), the child will also stop growing. Precocious puberty may be caused by pituitary tumors, other types of brain tumors, and very rarely by radiation therapy used to treat certain tumors.

Delayed adolescence will occur if a tumor has destroyed the ability of the pituitary to secrete the increased level of sexual hormones that should normally occur during adolescence. Tumors of the pineal gland, pituitary gland, and base of the brain, as well as radiation therapy, can cause delayed adolescence. Administering the appropriate hormones can correct the deficiency.

Disorders of Sexual Function

Several types of brain tumors may cause problems with sexual function. Pituitary tumors may cause impotence in males and loss of sexual drive as well as infertility in females. Tumors involving the frontal lobes can also cause personality changes that affect the sex drive. The change is usually a loss of interest in sex, but certain individuals will become much more sexually active.

Weight Loss and Obesity

Weight loss and appetite loss are common in patients with any type of cancer, but are especially likely in patients with brain tumors. If increased intracranial pressure occurs, weight loss will be even more dramatic because of nausea and vomiting associated with it. Radiation and chemotherapy will further increase weight loss, at least during the treatment period.

Some rare tumors involving the hypothalamus and thalamus cause a condition known as diencephalic syndrome. This results not only in weight loss, but also in complete absence of fat beneath the skin, giving it a very waxy appearance.

A few pituitary tumors secrete ACTH, a hormone that causes the body to release much more cortisone than usual. The cortisone causes increased appetite and weight gain. Usually, the increased fat is deposited in the abdomen, across the back of the shoulders, and in the face. The appearance of people with this condition is so characteristic that doctors refer to them as having a Cushingoid appearance, after Harvey Cushing, M.D., who first described the symptoms. Treatment of the pituitary tumor reduces cortisone levels in the body, though the affected person's appearance may never return to normal.

Abnormalities of Antidiuretic Hormone

Abnormally low levels of Antidiuretic Hormone (ADH) can occur if a tumor damages the pituitary, or if the gland was damaged by surgery or radiation used to treat a pituitary tumor. When this occurs, urine production increases dramatically, and body fluids are lost rapidly until severe dehydration occurs. This condition is called diabetes insipidus. When it occurs after pituitary damage, diabetes insipidus may require lifelong treatment with replacement hormone. It can also occur after surgery or injury involving other parts of the brain. In these cases, the condition will usually resolve on its own and does not require long-term treatment.

Excessive secretion of ADH occurs when the brain (specifically the hypothalamus) is slightly damaged and sends messages to the pituitary gland to increase ADH secretion. The affected person experiences weight gain and fluid retention. In severe cases, confusion and even seizures can result because the body retains so much water that the salt balance in the cells becomes upset. This condition is not limited to tumors in the region of the pituitary; it can be caused by any condition that increases intracranial pressure or irritates the brain. It can also occur after brain surgery of almost any type and is sometimes observed after a stroke.

Hypopituitarism

Hypopituitarism means that there is a deficiency (or even complete absence) of all pituitary hormone and releasing factor production. It generally results from almost complete destruction of the pituitary, sometimes as the result of surgery or radiation to remove a pituitary tumor. The symptoms are a combination of all of the deficiencies of the various hormones already discussed. Patients experience lethargy, mental changes, weight gain, fluid loss, and sexual dysfunction. The condition is treated by administering daily replacements of the various hormones.

OTHER SYMPTOMS OF BRAIN TUMORS

Although it does not occur frequently, brain tumors can sometimes cause symptoms that are confused with psychiatric illnesses. It is common for patients with undiagnosed brain tumors to have sleepiness,

lack of energy, and changes in mood that can be confused with depression. Other tumors can cause impaired mental function and
memory loss similar to that of Alzheimer's disease or senility. This is
particularly likely in patients with frontal or temporal lobe tumors.
These same tumors can also cause personality changes including increased aggression or anger, or bursts of sadness or weeping.

Rare tumors involving the temporal lobe can actually cause hallucinations. The affected person may hear strange sounds, or think that
they hear voices that aren't present. Parietal and occipital lobe tumors
can even cause visual hallucinations, although simple distorted vision
is far more common.

The Diagnosis of Brain Tumors

The diagnosis of any brain tumor requires that someone first of all become suspicious that one may exist. Once a doctor becomes suspicious, he or she will order studies to image the brain itself. Modern
CT and MRI scans (see chapter 4) can detect a mass as small as one-
third inch in diameter in many cases.

Depending upon the appearance and location of the mass, doctors
may be able to make an educated guess as to the type of tumor present. In the majority of cases, however, they will need to perform a
biopsy to determine exactly what type of tumor is present and to
grade its degree of severity (malignancy). This information is absolutely necessary to treat the tumor effectively.

IMAGING STUDIES OF THE BRAIN

A more detailed description of the various imaging studies can be
found in chapter 4. They are discussed briefly here simply to provide
an overview of the possible findings that each type of imaging can
provide for the diagnosis of brain tumor.

Standard CT scans can show large tumors, especially if there is a significant degree of swelling around the tumor. To effectively show most kinds of tumors, however, the CT scan must be performed with contrast, that is, an x-ray dye that binds to brain tissue is injected into a vein before the scan is performed. Using contrast, CT scan can effectively show most tumors in the cerebral hemispheres that are one-half inch or greater in diameter. They do not show tumors of the cerebellum or brain stem very well, however.

MRI scans are the diagnostic tool of choice. An MRI scan will detect tumors in size somewhat smaller than a CT scan can, and it can detect tumors of the cerebellum and brain stem quite effectively. The contrast media used in an MRI scan is also considered safer than that used in a CT scan, since it is less likely to cause either an allergic reaction or kidney problems. MRI scans are more difficult for the patient, however. Very large people may have trouble fitting into the scanner, while others find that the scanner causes them to feel claustrophobic. People who have had certain metal implants in their body, such as pacemakers, may not be able to have an MRI scan because of the strong magnetic field it generates.

PET scans generally do not provide as accurate a picture as MRI scans do, and the scarcity of the equipment involved means that few people will have access to a PET scanner anyway. PET scanners do provide some information about the metabolism of cells in the brain. Since many tumors have a high metabolism, PET scanners could theoretically be useful in diagnosing some tumors, but in the vast majority of cases, an MRI scan provides more information.

Radionuclide scans involve injecting short-lived radioactive material into a vein. The medication concentrates more highly in tumor or diseased tissue than in normal brain tissue, and this increased concentration can be detected by the scanner, which shows the tumor location. There are few situations in which a radionuclide scan is more accurate than an MRI scan, however.

SPECIAL DIAGNOSTIC STUDIES

Prior to the widespread availability of MRI and CT scans, there were a variety of complicated x-ray studies and other procedures used to detect brain tumors, none of which were particularly accurate. During this time exploratory surgery was sometimes needed to confirm that a tumor was even present. Today, exploratory surgery is rarely, if ever, indicated to diagnose the presence of a tumor. Once it is detected, a biopsy of the tumor is often required, however.

Lumbar puncture (spinal tap) is generally avoided in persons who may have a brain tumor because they may have increased intracranial pressure. However, tests of spinal fluid may identify tumor markers (substances that indicate the presence of a tumor) for a few types of rare tumors originating in the pineal gland. Unfortunately, most brain tumors have no tumor markers so the test is rarely indicated.

Arteriogram (injection of x-ray dye into the arteries of the brain) is not needed to diagnose brain tumors. In a few circumstances, the surgeon may request an arteriogram so that he or she can determine exactly where the blood supply of a tumor originates from or if the tumor involves one of the major arteries of the brain.

BRAIN BIOPSY

A biopsy is a surgical procedure used to remove a small amount of tumor tissue that can then be examined microscopically by a neuropathologist. Without this examination, it is impossible to accurately determine the type of tumor that is present and whether it is malignant or benign. If surgical removal of the tumor is planned, the biopsy is performed as part of the surgery. The surgeon will wait while the pathologist examines the tissue and proceed with the surgery if the tumor is what was anticipated.

When surgical removal is not planned, the biopsy may be performed through a small hole drilled in the skull. In these cases a procedure known as stereotaxic surgery is used. Stereotaxy provides a three-dimensional map of the brain. Prior to the procedure, a rigid metal frame is placed on the patient's head, and CT scans are used to determine the exact distance the tumor is located from several points on the frame. During surgery, a small hole, called a burr hole, is made in the patient's skull. The surgeon can then insert a special needle into the tumor to obtain a biopsy, using the frame as a reference point. If necessary, intraoperative x-ray, ultrasound, or other scanning devices can help pinpoint the tumor's location.

CHAPTER 12

Craniotomy and Surgery for Brain Tumors

Most people who have a brain tumor will require some type of surgery. When a benign tumor is located in an accessible area of the brain, complete surgical removal is often the only treatment necessary. Some malignant tumors may also be completely removed—if removal can be accomplished without causing severe neurological damage. Surgical removal alone will not cure a malignant tumor, however, since some tumor cells will have most likely invaded normal brain tissue.

Even partial removal of a malignant tumor can be beneficial. Partial removal provides an accurate diagnosis, reduces symptoms caused by the tumor, and leaves fewer tumor cells for other treatments to deal with. During surgery involving partial removal, implanted radiation seeds or chemotherapy beads may be inserted into the tumor site, providing a more effective treatment than could be obtained with standard chemotherapy or radiation.

Surgical removal of a brain tumor usually requires a craniotomy— removal of a portion of the skull to expose the brain. In certain cases, however, a craniotomy can be avoided. Tumors in certain locations, especially those near the pituitary gland, can be removed entirely without performing a craniotomy. For other tumors that are known to respond well to radiation or chemotherapy, surgery may consist of only a biopsy (removing a small piece of the tumor for examination). Many biopsies can now be performed using stereotactic techniques that require only a small hole drilled in the skull.

When a craniotomy is required, the preparations and general procedure are similar no matter where the actual tumor is located. The location chosen for the craniotomy, and the surgical techniques required for actual tumor removal, can be quite different depending upon the location of the tumor, but differences in these techniques will have little effect on the patient prior to surgery or during recovery.

The Preparation for Surgery

The preparations that occur before surgery are similar for all neurosurgical procedures involving a craniotomy. Increasingly, insurance companies and health maintenance organizations insist that patients not be admitted to the hospital until the day of their surgery. When this is the case, you will usually be asked to come to the hospital's outpatient department a few days before surgery for any necessary laboratory studies and to meet with an anesthesiologist about your surgery.

At this time the anesthesiologist will take a medical history and perform a limited physical examination. You will be advised of the risks of anesthesia (unless you have significant medical problems these are minimal) and told what the immediate postoperative plans will be. In some cases, this preoperative visit may not take place until the morning of surgery.

The morning of surgery, the surgeon or a member of his staff will discuss the surgical procedure in more detail, including all the risks and benefits of the procedure and any alternative treatments that are available. After all your questions are answered, you will be asked to sign a consent form, agreeing to the operation.

Obviously, the morning of surgery is not the best time to decide if you want to have surgery. Unfortunately, many patients don't really get a chance to have all their questions answered before this time. It is most important that the patient and their family make sure that they have had a chance to ask any questions they may have before the day of surgery. This often means you must take the initiative, scheduling an appointment (or asking for time during the surgeon's rounds if you're in the hospital) to discuss the surgery and all the various options. Neurosurgeons are busy people. If you don't ask for time to discuss the procedure, they will usually assume you have no questions. However, they will not be offended if you ask why they have chosen a certain treatment or want to ask exactly what the treatment involves.

One question most patients ask is whether their head will have to be shaved. For any craniotomy, that part of the head near the incision will have to be shaved since the hair contains bacteria that could cause infection. In some hospitals, an orderly or nurse will cut your hair and shave your head before you are taken to the operating room. In others, this will be done after you have been put to sleep. In either case, the nurses will save your hair if your request it. A wig manufacturer can use your own hair to make a natural looking wig that can be worn after surgery until your hair grows back (although this is rather expensive). If the surgery is simply a needle biopsy, only a small area of hair will be removed, while for transphenoidal procedures (see pages 190–191) hair removal is not necessary.

Most people expect to get a "preop" shot prior to surgery, and you may well receive one. With modern anesthesia, however, a preoperative shot is not necessary but rather is used only if you are nervous and need sedation. Because medications used for sedation can slow your breathing, the surgeon or anesthesiologist may prefer not to give a sedative to patients who have large tumors or increased intracranial pressure.

There are other medications given before surgery in many cases, but these will usually be administered through an intravenous line. For most patients undergoing a craniotomy for tumor removal, steroids are either started twenty-four hours prior to the operation or a single high dose is given just before surgery. An antibiotic is also administered intravenously just before surgery to help prevent any infection.

Once you arrive at the operating room, a nurse or anesthesiologist will start an intravenous (IV) line in one of your arms if one has not been started already. An automatic blood pressure cuff and electrocardiogram leads will also be placed. If your procedure is being performed under local anesthesia (some biopsies are done this way), you will be given some sedatives and pain medication through the IV before the start of the procedure. If you are having general anesthesia, you will breathe oxygen through a mask for a minute or two, and then be given anesthetics through the IV.

After you are put to sleep, a frame may be attached to your head to keep the skull immobile during surgery. The frame is attached with pins inserted through the skin. It causes no discomfort (obviously, you're asleep), but some patients notice the puncture marks after surgery and wonder where they came from.

Description of the Surgical Procedures

CRANIOTOMY

The actual surgical techniques involved in performing a craniotomy (removal of part of the skull) are generally the same no matter where the tumor is located. Only the location of the surgical incision differs depending upon exactly which part of the brain must be exposed for surgery. In general, exposure of the frontal lobes requires an incision across the top of the skull, from above one ear to the other ear. Exposure of the parietal lobe is done through a C- or U-shaped incision above and behind the ear. Exposure of the cerebellum, occipital lobes, and posterior portion of the temporal lobes is done through a linear or slightly curved incision behind the ear.

After the skin incision has been made and any bleeding stopped, the surgeon will scrape away the muscles and connective tissue that cover the skull. A special drill is used to make several small holes (called burr holes) through the skull, and then a saw is used to cut through the skull between the holes until a roughly circular piece of skull has been removed. If the craniotomy is being performed at the back of the skull, where bone is thicker, a special high-speed drill may be used to scrape away the bone in that area, rather than removing a single piece of the skull. Replacement of the skull is not necessary in these areas, because the thick muscles at the base of the skull provide adequate protection for the brain.

Once the portion of skull has been removed, the surgeon will then make an incision through the tough meningeal membranes (called the dura) that cover the brain itself. After these membranes have been opened, the brain itself is exposed. In the case of a meningioma or other tumor that actually involves the dura, the section containing the tumor is completely removed, leaving a large hole in the meningeal membranes. The surgeon will then remove a piece of connective tissue from another part of the body, usually from the muscles of the hip, to "patch" the hole in the meningeal membranes. In other cases, the dura is simply sewn closed at the end of surgery.

Benign tumors usually have a covering that clearly separates them from healthy brain tissue. When benign tumors are located near the surface of the brain, they can often be dissected free from the surrounding brain tissue and removed in one piece. The surgeon must proceed carefully to avoid damage to surrounding healthy brain tissue and to identify and cauterize (burn) each of the blood vessels going into the tumor.

Malignant tumors do not have a clear border between themselves and surrounding brain tissue. In these cases the surgeon will arbitrarily remove the obvious tumor along with some apparently healthy brain tissue near the edge of the tumor. The amount of tissue actually removed depends upon the type of tumor, the tumor's size, and how critical the nearby brain areas are.

When tumors are located deep within the brain, the surgeon must dissect through normal brain tissue to reach the tumor. In many of these cases, a stereotactic procedure (see pages 193–195) is used to localize the tumor. In other cases, the surgeon may use intraoperative ultrasound, or even CT and MRI scans developed especially for use in the operating room, to localize the tumor. Once the tumor has been exposed, it is removed as completely as possible. Obviously, it is much more difficult to completely remove a tumor located deep within the brain than one close to the surface.

The surgeon may employ any of several tools to actually remove the tumor, including an old-fashioned scalpel. For smaller tumors, the surgeon may perform all the actual tumor removal using an operating microscope, allowing a clear view of the separation between the tumor and normal brain tissue. Operating lasers may be used instead of the traditional scalpel and cautery. The laser generates immense heat focused on a small area, destroying the tumor by vaporizing it a bit at a time. Large tumors are often removed by an ultrasonic aspirator. This tool uses high frequency vibrations to break up the tumor into small pieces that are removed by suction.

It is important to remember that while all these devices make tumor removal safer and more complete, none of them are "miracles." They cannot remove every malignant cell from normal brain tissue. No one of them is perfect for every application. Each has its particular strengths and weaknesses and can prove most useful for certain kinds of tumors.

After the tumor has been removed, the surgeon carefully inspects the brain to insure that there is no bleeding. The meningeal membranes are then sewn closed, the portion of skull that has been re-moved is replaced, and the skin is sewn shut.

After removal of a small tumor in the meningeal membranes or on the surface of the brain, most people are awake within a few hours following surgery. In the case of larger tumors, or tumors located deep within the brain, the surgeon may prefer to keep the patient heavily sedated and on a mechanical ventilator for hours or even a day or two after surgery. Often, the surgeon will perform a CT or MRI scan the day after surgery to make sure there is no significant bleeding or swelling in the brain. If the surgery was extensive, the surgeon may also place a pressure monitor through the skull so he or she can watch for any increased intracranial pressure.

Although 95 percent of patients will have no major problems following a craniotomy, complications can occur, especially if the surgery involves a very large or deeply located tumor. If there is post-operative bleeding, a repeat surgical procedure may be required to re-move the clotted blood and stop the bleeding. This procedure is usually much quicker and simpler than the original surgery because dissection of the tumor is not required. Swelling of the brain is also possible but can usually be controlled with medications, fluid restric-tion, and mechanical ventilation.

With any craniotomy, infection is a low but ever-present risk. If the infection involves the brain or meningeal membranes lining the brain, it is diagnosed by analyzing spinal fluid and treated with an-tibiotics. If the infection involves the skin or skull bone, it may be nec-essary to surgically remove the infected tissue and reclose the wound by means of a skin graft.

Other complications that can occur after a craniotomy are gener-ally related to the damage to parts of the brain near where the tumor was located. Complications are treated similarly to those of a stroke patient: physical therapy and occupational therapy are used to restore as much function as possible.

TRANSPHENOIDAL SURGICAL PROCEDURES

The pituitary gland actually "hangs" down below the brain, being located in a small opening in the base of the skull that is surrounded by fairly thin bone. This area is above and behind the sinuses at the back of the nose. By operating through the nasal cavities and sinuses, the pituitary gland can be reached without requiring a craniotomy. The procedure is called transphenoidal surgery because the operation takes place through the sphenoid sinus, the sinus that lies just in front of the pituitary gland.

Transphenoidal surgery is performed via an incision made in the upper gum, under the lip. Often an otolaryngologist (ear, nose, and throat surgeon) will perform the initial exposure, with the neurosurgeon then performing actual tumor removal. Some neurosurgeons perform the entire procedure themselves.

After making the initial incision, the surgeon dissects a tunnel below the nasal cartilage and above the roof of the mouth until the thin case of bone surrounding the pituitary gland is reached. A high-speed drill is then used to remove this bone, and an operating microscope placed so that the surgeon can inspect the pituitary gland. Using small suctions and spoon-shaped instruments, the surgeon removes the tumor from the gland. Recovery after a transphenoidal procedure usually takes four to five days. The nose will be packed with gauze for three or four days after surgery, and the area is usually sore for a week or two. Patients can usually return to work in about four weeks.

An alternate technique that is now used more frequently replaces the operating microscope with an endoscope. Endoscopes are tubes containing lenses and fiberoptic lights that allow the surgeon a closer view of the gland compared to the standard operating microscope. Openings in the tube allow special instruments to be passed into the area of operation without obstructing the surgeon's view. The endoscope is threaded through the nostril so a surgical incision above the lip and dissection beneath the nasal cartilage is not required.

The results with endoscopic surgery are about the same as with standard transphenoidal surgery, but it requires a shorter postoperative stay in the hospital. It also eliminates the need for nasal packing after surgery, resulting in less pain and facial swelling.

Transphenoidal surgery is usually an elective operation, scheduled several days in advance. In a few patients it becomes an emergency procedure, however. This occurs if a large pituitary tumor outgrows its blood supply resulting in a stroke of the pituitary gland. The gland enlarges rapidly as the tissue swells, causing a severe headache, double vision, and eventually blindness. This is known as pituitary apoplexy and requires emergency surgery to prevent permanent blindness.

ACOUSTIC NEUROMA SURGERY

Removal of acoustic neuromas requires a somewhat different approach because of the location of the tumor and because the surgeon will try to avoid damage to the cranial nerves that are located near the tumor. The nerve nearest the acoustic nerve is the facial nerve, which carries muscle impulses to the face. If the facial nerve is damaged, the patient will experience weakness or paralysis on one side of the face, which can prove quite disfiguring. For this reason, electrical monitoring of the facial nerve is usually performed during acoustic neuroma surgery.

In cases when the surgeon will attempt to save the acoustic nerve (which carries hearing from the ear to the brain), a second monitoring device will be used to measure evoked potentials. This device measures brain wave changes that are caused when a sound reaches the eardrum and is monitored during the entire surgical procedure. If the evoked potentials weaken, the surgeon will know that he is putting too much pressure on the nerve and can change the technique being used to remove the tumor.

The incision for exposure of an acoustic neuroma is made over the thick bone just behind the ear (called the mastoid process). It is made in a straight line and is usually about three inches long. After making the incision, the surgeon must dissect through the thick muscles that attach to the skull in this area. Some surgeons then remove a piece of the skull as would be done for a craniotomy, while others use a special drill to shave away the skull in this region until the meningeal membranes are exposed.

After the meningeal membranes have been opened, the surgeon will again use a drill to open the bony canal that the acoustic nerve follows between the brain and the ear. An operating microscope is used to allow the surgeon to identify each of the nerves in the area. Once the acoustic nerve has been identified, the tumor is dissected free of the nerve in an attempt to spare the nerve and save the patient's hearing on that side.

If the tumor is large, it may have to be removed in several pieces. In this case the surgeon will make every attempt to identify and save the facial nerve so that muscle function to the face remains intact. It is usually impossible to save the acoustic nerve in this situation, and the ear on that side will be deaf after surgery (generally, patients with large tumors are already deaf on the affected side).

Although a cure is expected after removal of an acoustic neuroma, the surgery does not come without risk. As with any surgical procedure, the possibility of infection—although low—is always present. Postoperative bleeding or infarction in the cerebellum can occur, requiring an immediate reoperation to reduce swelling near the brain stem. It is also possible for a patient to develop hydrocephalus after this surgery, but usually this complication is only temporary. Leaking of cerebrospinal fluid through the area of surgery is also possible and usually will require a reoperation to repair the meningeal membranes.

Despite every attempt to identify and spare cranial nerves in the area, it is possible that some of them will be damaged during the surgery. If this occurs, the patient may experience partial paralysis of the face or difficulty swallowing. With physical therapy and over time these problems will often disappear, but in a few cases they prove permanent. Finally, a few people experience a persistent headache after surgery for acoustic neuroma. Usually the headache appears to be caused by the muscles at the base of the skull that were damaged during the surgery; it typically will respond to physical therapy or injections of cortisone into the muscles.

STEREOTACTIC SURGERY AND SPECIAL PROCEDURES

Stereotactic surgery is used to allow surgeons to place a needle or small device with precision in a certain location without having to perform a complete craniotomy. The technique constructs a very accurate three-dimensional map of an individual's brain, which can then enable doctors to measure the direction and distance of any brain structure from specific points on a frame attached to the skull.

Stereotactic surgical techniques provide remarkable accuracy. Using modern systems, a surgeon can place a needle into the brain to within an accuracy of 1 mm (about ⅛ inch). The procedure may be used during open craniotomy for surgery, but currently is most commonly used to obtain a needle biopsy of a tumor so that craniotomy is not necessary. Stereotactic localization is also used to perform laser microsurgery, administer high doses of external radiation, and to implant radioactive seeds in the brain.

Stereotactic Biopsy
The first step in a stereotactic procedure is application of the stereotactic frame. The frame is usually a ring-shaped structure attached to the skull with four pins. The areas where the frame will be attached (usually to each temple near the forehead and two areas near the back of the head) will be shaved in a one-inch square and scrubbed using a soap and iodine solution. The surgeon will inject a local anesthetic into each area to numb the skin and muscles in that location.

The surgeon will then position the ring and fix it in place using four steel pins that pierce the skin. This part of the procedure is painless.

It is important to keep your eyes closed during the procedure so that the pins don't "trap" any of the forehead muscles, which could keep you from closing your eyes once the frame is in place. Although the location of the frame may vary slightly depending upon the location of the tumor, it will usually circle the head just above the eyebrows.

Once the frame has been attached to your head, a second ring or arch, called a localizing ring, is attached to the frame. You will then undergo a CT scan (see chapter 4) with the frame in place. This scan takes thirty minutes or more, since an additional number of "slices" must be taken. After the scan a computer will determine the exact distance between certain points on the frame and the tumor (or vital structures near the tumor). The computer then converts the distances into sets of coordinates measured as direction and distance from points on the frame and localizing ring.

After this has been done, you will be taken to the operating room with the frame still in place. The operating room will have a special operating table with attachments for the stereotactic frame so that it can't move during surgery. You will be given sedative medications but usually not put entirely to sleep during the procedure.

Your head will be scrubbed again and more hair may need to be shaved. The surgeons will place sterile sheets and drapes so that the top of your head is exposed but the rest of your body is covered. The anesthesiologist will clip the sheets so that they are away from your face, and he or she will be able to talk to you during the entire procedure.

Just as during the placement of the stereotactic frame, local anesthetic will be used to numb the skin of your scalp. The surgeon will make a small incision about an inch long, and then use a drill to make a small hole through the skull. You will hear the noise and may feel vibrations from the drill, but won't experience any pain during this part of the procedure.

After the hole has been drilled, the neurosurgeons will place an arch-shaped device to the stereotactic frame. Alternatively, they may use a localizer arm (a jointed arm that can be precisely positioned from a single point on the stereotactic frame). Using computer-generated coordinates from the CT scan, the biopsy needle is set in the arch or arm and advanced to the exact depth required. Since the brain itself has no pain nerves, you will not feel the needle at all. The material obtained from the needle is sent to the pathology lab to be stained and examined microscopically.

After the needle is removed, the skin is closed using a few stitches, a small bandage is placed, and the frame removed. Usually the pin insertion sites do not need to be stitched; they are simply covered with a band aid. Immediately after the operation you will be taken to the recovery room. You will be kept in the recovery room for an hour or more after surgery so that nurses can assess your condition frequently. Every few minutes, the surgeon or a nurse will ask you to move your arms and legs and answer a few questions. This is simply to insure that no bleeding is occurring within the brain itself.

After this you will be sent back to your room and usually kept in the hospital overnight for observation. You will be asked to sleep with the head of your bed elevated and to limit the amount of fluid you drink in order to minimize the risk of brain swelling. In some cases, you will be asked not to get out of bed or walk for twenty-four hours following the procedure.

Although the surgeon may get a preliminary biopsy report immediately after surgery, the special stains required by the pathologist to accurately assess the tumor take several days to prepare. The surgeon may not be able to discuss further treatment with you until after discussing the results with the pathologist.

SHUNTS

Placement of a shunt is not actually a procedure to treat the brain tumor itself, but is often required to treat hydrocephalus. A shunt is a plastic tube that connects one of the ventricles of the brain to another part of the body. The extra fluid can pass through the shunt, thus relieving this extra pressure on the brain. The most common type of shunt is tunnelled under the skin to the abdomen, allowing the cerebrospinal fluid to pass into the abdominal cavity where it can be absorbed.

The procedure is usually performed under general anesthesia following preparations similar to a craniotomy. Only a small burr hole is required for the shunt catheter to enter the ventricle; a complete craniotomy is not required. The tube is then tunnelled under the skin until it reaches the abdomen.

Symptoms usually improve immediately after the insertion of a shunt. Doctors will monitor the shunt to make sure it remains open, but most people can go home from the hospital in a day or two.

Advances in Brain Surgery

INTRAOPERATIVE MRI

Magnetic resonance imaging is the standard method used to detect tumors in the brain, but the complicated equipment required and high magnetic fields generated usually mean that the MRI must be located in a building separate from the rest of the hospital. Recent advances have allowed the development of an MRI that uses two doughnut-shaped devices to generate the magnetic field. This allows the patient's head to be accessible to the surgeon while an MRI scan is obtained.

MRI scanners allow direct intraoperative evaluation of a tumor during surgery. The most common application for this technology is for needle biopsy and similar procedures, but by using special instruments a surgeon can perform a complete craniotomy and tumor resection under MRI guidance. Currently the equipment is still under investigation and available in only a few medical centers. Its cost will limit its usefulness to a few specific types of tumor surgery even when it becomes increasingly available. Indications for using the equipment will probably include recurrent low-grade tumors where the tumor margin is not obvious, and tumors located in difficult to expose areas of the brain stem and cerebellum.

ENDOSCOPIC SURGERY FOR SKULL BASE TUMORS

Tumors located near the base of the skull are very difficult to expose surgically because of the thickness of the skull in this area and the location of many vital structures nearby. Surgeons have recently begun using the endoscopic equipment developed for transphenoidal pituitary surgery to attempt to reach these tumors. The technique is now becoming accepted for other tumors in the pituitary area, such as epidermoid tumors, meningiomas, and craniopharyngiomas.

FRAMELESS STERFOTACTIC SURGERY

Currently, stereotactic frames provide the most accurate method for a surgeon to localize deep structures within the brain. However, to use these systems a frame must be applied to the head, the patient must then undergo a CT or MRI scan with the frame in place, and the frame must remain in place during the surgical procedure. The frame itself can restrict the surgeon's choice of location for the craniotomy. The systems are extremely accurate, however, allowing the surgeon to place an instrument within an accuracy of 1 mm.

Several frameless systems for stereotactic localization are currently under development. These systems still require a preoperative MRI or CT scan, but don't require a large frame to be placed on the patient's head, thus allowing the surgeon more freedom of access during the actual procedure. All these systems use computers attached to special instruments to determine exactly where an instrument is placed within the brain. Currently all have limitations, but some form of frameless stereotactic surgery should be widely available within two to five years. Though their accuracy is slightly less than that of standard stereotactic frame systems, they are still accurate to within 3 or 4 mm.

CHAPTER 13

Other Treatments

Most malignant brain tumors cannot be removed completely during surgery because they have already spread into surrounding tissues. Some additional form of treatment will always be needed to prevent these tumors from recurring. Nonsurgical treatments may be the only option when surgery isn't possible because of the tumor's location or type.

Radiation therapy is a mainstay for brain tumor treatment. It is sometimes used before surgery to help "shrink" a tumor, but is frequently employed following surgery to kill any remaining tumor cells in the brain. New techniques including implanted radiation seeds and highly focused radiation beams have made radiation therapy more effective while at the same time limiting its side effects.

Chemotherapy is generally not as effective against brain tumors as against other types of cancer, but it may still be valuable for treating certain types of brain tumors. As with radiation therapy, there have been significant advances in brain tumor chemotherapy. Research into new anticancer drugs is continually improving the outcomes of several types of brain tumors. There are also new methods of administering chemotherapy that can enhance its effectiveness, while minimizing the side effects associated with these drugs.

When a brain tumor does recur, a second surgical removal is sometimes attempted. Unfortunately, repeat operations in the same area are technically more difficult and less likely to be successful than the original surgery. Chemotherapy is often used to treat recurrent tumors, especially mid-grade tumors. Radiation, particularly focused beam radiations such as gamma knife radiation, are treatment mainstays for recurrent tumors.

It is important to remember that every person and every tumor is unique. Be careful not to assume that the "miraculous" recovery some people experienced after a certain treatment will happen to you. Deciding the best treatment for a particular situation must take many factors into account. Older people and those with significant medical illness may not be able to withstand the effects of certain chemotherapy or surgical procedures, for example. A tumor's location may mean that surgery would very likely destroy important brain functions, while another person's tumor that differs in location by a mere inch may be easily removed. A large tumor is more difficult to remove completely and may be considered inoperable simply because of its size.

All these factors plus many others influence the physician's decisions concerning which treatment is best for a particular person's tumor. It is important, however, that you explore all your options and reach an informed decision that is right for you. If you aren't comfortable understanding why a certain treatment isn't available to you or why another treatment is being recommended, get a second opinion. It's also important to ask your doctor if there may be treatments that are not being offered to you because of your insurance company's rules or standards. In many cases, you can appeal these rules to gain access to a treatment that was denied originally.

Radiation Therapy

Most brain tumors are quite sensitive to radiation. For many years, beams of high power x-rays or gamma rays aimed at tumors from ex-

ternal sources have been used to treat brain tumors. This type of therapy, called standard radiotherapy, is given in separate treatments every
few days for a period of several weeks to two months.

In some cases, other types of radiation may be more effective or
cause fewer side effects. Small seeds of radioactive material can be implanted directly into the tumor, a technique called interstitial radiation or brachytherapy. In other cases, high-energy radiation is tightly
focused onto a small area of the brain. This technique avoids expos-
ing normal brain tissue to radiation, but requires that the beam be directed precisely in the area of the tumor. To accomplish this, frame
and CT-directed measurements, as would be used for stereotactic
surgery (see chapter 12), are necessary to provide an exact guide for
the radiation beam.

STANDARD RADIATION THERAPY

Radiation is a general term used to describe several types of high energy beams. There are two broad categories of radiation: particle radiation and electromagnetic radiation. Electromagnetic radiation is
generally what we think of as "pure" energy. It is the same type of energy that makes heat and light, only much more powerful. X-rays and
gamma rays are the two types of electromagnetic radiation commonly
used to treat tumors. Most people who have radiation treatments for
cancer are actually receiving high energy x-rays.

Particle radiation consists of parts of atoms (electrons, neutrons,
protons) moving at very high speeds. This is the type of radiation that
we usually think of when we talk about nuclear power. Beta particles,
which consist of electrons moving at high speeds, are the least ener-
getic type of particle radiation but are still more powerful than x-rays
or gamma rays. Alpha particles, which contain neutrons, contain ever
higher energy than Beta particles. Most implanted radiation seeds
give off particle radiation.

In either case, the principle behind radiation therapy is simple.
High energy from the radiation is absorbed by tissues in the area

irradiated, where it causes damage. Fast-growing cells (such as most tumor cells) are sensitive to radiation and easily destroyed. Slow-growing cells (normal brain cells are very slow growing) are more re-sistant to radiation and less likely to be destroyed.

When radiation is used to treat brain tumors (or other tumors for that matter), the radiation is focused on the area of the tumor, but some radiation will inevitably strike normal brain tissue. In fact, the radiation must include the normal brain tissue around the tumor, since this is the area where microscopic tumor cells are invading the brain. Even though normal brain cells are fairly resistant to radiation, there may be some damage to the brain in this area.

Standard radiation therapy is administered in many small doses over a period of time. For some types of tumors this may mean sev-eral doses each a week apart, while others tumors respond best to a smaller amount of radiation every day for several weeks. Each treat-ment may take anywhere from a few minutes to half an hour.

In order to focus the radiation onto the location of the tumor, it is important that your head be kept completely still during the radia-tion treatment. Since it is impossible for anyone to hold perfectly still during the entire radiation treatment, a mold of your head will usu-ally be made before your first radiation treatment. This requires a plaster cast to be made, which is then converted into a plastic shell that fits your head snugly. During each radiation treatment the shell is fixed in place on a radiation grid so that your head doesn't move.

Standard radiation causes several side effects. The most important of these is swelling in the area of the brain being treated. Most of this swelling results from tumor cells dying, so in a way it is a good side effect, but if left untreated the swelling can cause pressure on other structures in the brain. Most people undergoing brain radiation will have to take Decadron® or another type of cortisone to minimize swelling during the treatments.

Radiation will also cause hair loss in the area of the skull that the x-ray passes through. Hair loss doesn't usually begin until about ten days after treatments have started, although it may happen sooner or later depending upon the amount of radiation given at each treatment. Hair loss can be permanent, but most people will have at least some hair return in the affected area within two to three months after treatments have been completed.

Other common side effects of radiation are skin irritation and redness, nausea sometimes accompanied by vomiting, fatigue, and generally feeling ill. Some people develop short-term memory loss or feel that their thinking is becoming slowed during the period when they are undergoing radiation. Many of these side effects can be controlled with medications, so be certain to tell the radiation oncologist (the doctor who directs radiation therapy) if you experience them. These symptoms will usually clear up within six weeks after radiation therapy is completed.

IMPLANTED RADIATION

In some cases, seeds of radioactive material can be placed into the brain around a tumor site. This has the advantage of delivering high-energy radiation to the tumor without the radiation having to pass through normal tissue. Of course, it has the disadvantage of requiring surgery with the potential risk of infection and other complications.

If a craniotomy is being performed to remove most of the tumor, the radioactive material can be implanted easily at that time. If a craniotomy is not being performed, the radioactive material can be implanted using stereotactic surgery. When stereotactic procedures are used for radiation implantation, the procedure is almost exactly like that described for stereotactic biopsy (see chapter 12), except that the frames are applied and the CT scan performed the day before the procedure. This is necessary so that the doctors have time to calculate exactly where to place the radioactive seeds and how many will be needed for treatment.

In most cases, the actual surgical procedure involves implanting small, hollow catheters or tubes. A day or two after surgery, technicians from the radiation therapy department will load the radioactive seeds into the catheters. This process is entirely painless—they simply slip the seeds a premeasured distance into the catheters that are already in place. Afterwards, a repeat CT scan is performed to insure the seeds are placed exactly where they should be to provide the highest dose of radiation to the tumor—and the least amount to normal brain tissue.

Usually the radioactive seeds are left in the catheters for five to seven days. During this time you will be under "radiation precautions." The actual amount of radiation used is small, but there are very strict government regulations that must be followed to limit its potential exposure to other people. Pregnant women and children under the age of eighteen will not be allowed to visit while the radioactive seeds are in place. Every day or two, a radiation safety officer will measure the amount of radiation being given off to make sure there is no danger to other people. You may even be asked to use disposable utensils when you eat, or may have a lead-lined shield placed around your bed.

While the precautions may seem intimidating, there is actually not a great deal of radiation involved. The main purpose of the precautions is to protect health care workers who are exposed to patients with radiation implants day after day for years. Once the seeds and catheters have been removed, your body does not remain radioactive, and you will not emit any other radiation. After that time, nothing that you touch or otherwise come in contact with will become contaminated with radioactivity.

Removing the radioactive seeds is simple and almost painless. A radiation oncologist or technician will remove the seeds from the catheters. A detecting instrument will be used to make sure that all the seeds have been removed and no radioactivity remains. Once this is completed, the radiation precautions are over and you will have no restrictions.

After the radioactive seeds are removed, the neurosurgeon removes the catheters using local anesthesia to numb the skin around each one. Each catheter opening will usually require a single stitch to close it up, although sometimes a simple bandage is all that is required. Even if no stitches are needed, you will be told not to allow your head to get wet for two or three days. This is simply a precaution to avoid infection. If stitches are used, they will be removed in about seven days.

FOCUSED BEAM RADIATION (GAMMA KNIFE OR RADIOSURGERY)

The equipment needed to deliver very high-dose radiation in a tightly focused beam was developed in the late 1960s and early 1970s. Focused beam radiation has been used since that time but has become infinitely more effective since it was combined with the same stereotactic (meaning to accurately determine where a point is in three dimensions) techniques used to localize tumors accurately for surgery.

Focused beam radiation offers advantages in certain situations. Because a very narrow radiation beam is concentrated on a small area within the brain, a high dose of radiation can be administered without fear of damaging surrounding brain tissue. Modern focusing equipment is so specific that an area as small as a one-quarter-inch cube can be heavily irradiated while only a small amount of radiation reaches the surrounding brain tissue. When a situation requires it, stereotactic techniques can also be used to accurately give several small radiation doses over a period of weeks. These treatments are employed not only for tumors, but also to treat arteriovenous malformations and certain chronically painful conditions.

In either case, the technique provides the advantage of minimizing the amount of radiation absorbed by normal brain tissue, while maximizing the amount delivered to the area containing the tumor. Because the focused beam doesn't deliver significant amounts of radiation to other parts of the brain, even patients who have been treated previously with standard radiation can undergo focused radiation treatments.

By comparison, standard radiation therapy delivers high energy x-rays to both the tumor and the surrounding brain tissue. The radiation is given in small doses over several weeks, theoretically allowing normal brain tissue to recover from radiation damage while the more sensitive tumor cells are slowly destroyed. Standard radiation is especially effective when microscopic tumor cells have grown into normal brain tissue, and in such cases is more appropriate than focused beam radiation.

Focused beam radiation uses either a modified linear accelerator or a cobalt-60 machine as the radiation source. In the most common technique, very high energy gamma radiation from radioactive cobalt-60 is used. The equipment that focuses the radiation is referred to as a gamma knife at most centers, but some centers refer to the technique as radiosurgery.

An actual gamma knife machine contains about two hundred small pieces of cobalt, the source of the gamma rays. The cobalt is located in a thickly shielded machine capable of focusing individual gamma ray beams into a single point, called the focal point. Gamma rays are extremely intense at the focal point but much less intense only a fraction of an inch away from the focal point.

This equipment is capable of generating enough radiation during a single treatment to completely destroy all the cells in the selected area. For this reason, focused beam radiation is most effective when used to destroy localized tumors. It can be used not only for malignant tumors, but also for benign tumors located in areas that would be difficult to reach using surgery. Very often, an obvious tumor is destroyed by focused beam radiation, and then the surrounding brain receives standard radiation therapy in an attempt to destroy invading tumor cells.

Radiosurgery requires the combined efforts of a neurosurgeon, radiologist, and radiation oncologist. As with other stereotactic procedures, a lightweight aluminum frame is affixed to your head using local anesthesia by the neurosurgeon, after which a CT or MRI scan is obtained by the radiologist. The scan is used to calculate the specific lo-cation of the tumor, and the radiation oncologist determines the exact amount and type of radiation the tumor should receive.

During a gamma knife treatment, the stereotactic head frame is fixed inside the machine. Using the CT scan, doctors will program the machine's software to accurately place the focal point on the exact part(s) of the brain that should receive the treatment. Usually several different "shots" of gamma rays are required because the focal point is smaller than the area requiring treatment. The entire procedure usually takes from forty-five minutes to an hour. Afterwards, the frame is removed and the patient returns to their hospital room for overnight observation. In some cases, the entire procedure is done on an outpatient basis.

There is no pain during or after focused beam radiation therapy. Some people will experience swelling in the part of the brain that un-derwent treatment and require cortisone therapy just as they would with standard radiation. If the area being treated is small, however, this is often not necessary. Of course, if the area of treatment contains vital brain structures, there could be permanent loss of function of that area. If this is possible, doctors will know about it and discuss this possibility with you before treatment.

Focused radiation is frequently used to treat metastatic brain tu-mors originating from cancer in other parts of the body, and also to treat primary brain tumors that have recurred. In these situations, the gamma knife procedure can be as effective as surgery without expos-ing the patient to surgical risks and recovery. It is also used as an al-ternative to surgery for certain benign tumors such as meningiomas and acoustic neuromas. About 90 percent of meningiomas will stop growing after gamma knife treatment, and some reports indicate that 95 percent of acoustic neuromas actually shrink after gamma knife treatment.

The results of radiosurgery are not apparent immediately. Benign tumors may show no change other than they've stopped growing.

Malignant tumors may disappear completely over a few months. For most tumors, a repeat CT or MRI scan will be obtained three months after the gamma knife procedure to determine what affects the treatment has had on the tumor.

Chemotherapy

Chemotherapy basically consists of chemicals that poison tumor cells. As with radiation therapy, in theory the tumor cells are more sensitive to the chemicals than are healthy cells. In reality, certain tumors are sensitive only to certain chemotherapy agents, and some tumors are not sensitive to any of the drugs. Doctors will know from experience the types of drugs that are most likely to be effective against each type of brain tumor.

Most types of chemotherapy work by damaging the DNA of cells that are actively reproducing. Since tumor cells divide more often compared to most of the body's other cells, chemotherapy should damage many more tumor cells overall. The damage may prevent the two daughter cells from reproducing, or may make them unable to function properly, resulting in their death.

Other types of chemotherapy can kill certain cancer cells directly or prevent them from dividing. This type of chemotherapy takes advantage of the differences between certain tumor cells and normal cells. Some tumors are very sensitive to certain hormones, for example, and will stop dividing if the hormone is present.

There are currently over forty chemotherapeutic drugs available for use in the U.S., while a dozen more are under study or currently being used in Europe. Depending on the type of tumor involved, chemotherapy may be the lone treatment, can be used after surgery, or used in addition to radiation therapy. Recurrent brain tumors are often treated with chemotherapy, either alone or in addition to radiation therapy. Chemotherapy is also used to treat brain tumors in very young children since exposing the developing brain to radiation therapy is likely to cause long-term problems.

Administering effective chemotherapy for brain tumors is more difficult than administering chemotherapy for cancers in other parts of the body for several reasons. Most importantly, many brain tumors are not very sensitive to the commonly used chemotherapy agents. For this reason, chemotherapy for brain tumors usually requires a combination of several different chemotherapy drugs. Administering small doses of several drugs—each of which damages tumor cells in a different way—can be much more effective than a high dose of a single drug.

Additionally, the blood–brain barrier (see chapter 2) prevents certain types of chemotherapy chemicals from even reaching brain tissue. Some chemotherapy protocols add medications that disrupt the blood–brain barrier temporarily so that the chemotherapy can reach the brain. In other cases, new techniques have been developed to allow the chemotherapy drug to avoid the blood–brain barrier. These include injecting the drug into an artery going to the brain, delivering the drug directly into the cerebrospinal fluid, or surgically placing drug-saturated sponges into the area of the tumor.

Some treatments also include drugs that help the chemotherapy agents reach the tumor in greater concentration. Still other drugs may enhance radiation treatments by sensitizing tumor cells to radiation damage. Finally, although not strictly considered chemotherapy, some medications, such as cortisone, are often included with chemotherapy to minimize any damaging effects the drugs may have.

STANDARD CHEMOTHERAPY

The blood–brain barrier (see chapter 2) prevents most toxins from entering the brain. While this is an important protective barrier in healthy individuals, for those with tumors it prevents many chemotherapy agents from penetrating into the brain. There are several chemotherapy drugs that readily cross the blood–brain barrier, however, and these provide the mainstay of chemotherapy for brain tumors.

Research is also providing insight regarding ways of temporarily disrupting the blood–brain barrier so that chemotherapy can reach the brain. These involve either giving medications—such as mannitol—that make the barrier temporarily ineffective, or by injecting chemotherapy agents in high concentrations directly into arteries that provide blood flow to the tumor. In other cases, the drugs may be administered directly into the cerebrospinal fluid.

When treating brain tumors, combinations of several chemotherapy drugs given together usually elicit better results than any single chemotherapy drug. Combination therapy may work better because the different drugs have an additive effect on tumor cells; the two drugs together may kill the cell when either drug alone would cause only mild damage. It may also work because the different cells within the tumor have different sensitivities to the drugs: one drug kills some cells while another drug kills different cells. Additionally, combining drugs with different side effects means a higher total dose of chemotherapy can be given without the patient enduring severe side effects.

In general, chemotherapy is most effective against rapidly growing, highly malignant tumors. It is not effective against slow-growing, benign tumors. Exactly which drugs are most effective varies considerably depending upon the exact nature of the tumor. Every year new research reveals slightly better combinations of chemotherapy for different kinds of tumors.

Currently, chemotherapy appears to be most useful against glial cell tumors such as malignant astrocytomas and glioblastomas. Several clinical studies have shown that patients with astrocytoma or glioblastoma multiforme who receive chemotherapy, in addition to surgery or radiation, live almost twice as long as those who don't receive chemotherapy. Unfortunately, chemotherapy is less successful against recurrent glial tumors.

The number and frequency of each treatment depends on the drug combination being used. Some chemotherapy drugs can be taken by mouth, but most must be injected directly into a vein. If only a few treatments will be required, a nurse will usually start an IV line in the hand or arm to give the medication. If the chemotherapy is going to require many small doses, it may be necessary to surgically insert a device that allows the chemotherapy to be administered directly into a large vein.

A Port-a-Cath® is one of the most common methods used to provide long-term access to a vein, and many patients have this type of device inserted so that chemotherapy can be given more easily. The Port-a-Cath is implanted beneath the skin just below the collarbone. Its placement requires a minor surgical procedure under local anesthesia, and takes place in the operating room. Only a small incision is required, and there are no tubes visible outside the body. The injection port can be felt as a lump under the skin about the size of a stack of four or five quarters.

Once it is in place, chemotherapy can be given right into the Port-a-Cath without requiring an IV to be started for each treatment. The Port-a-Cath can also be used to give IV fluids or obtain blood samples whenever they are needed. The Port-a-Cath is removed when it is no longer required—usually a month or so after the last chemotherapy treatment.

Side Effects of Chemotherapy

Because chemotherapy kills all dividing cells, it affects normal tissues to some degree. Which normal tissues are most affected will vary depending upon the individual chemotherapy drug. In general, though, tissues that normally maintain a high growth rate such as the bone marrow (which produces blood cells), the linings of the intestines, and hair follicles are the most severely affected.

Damage to the bone marrow causes a fall in the white blood cell (cells that fight infection) count. The white blood cell counts reach their lowest point between seven and fourteen days after a chemotherapy treatment. Depending upon the type of chemotherapy being used, the white cell count may improve within a few days or remain low for several weeks. Some chemotherapeutic agents such as BCNU, which is commonly used in brain tumors, can damage the stem cells (the cells that give rise to the white blood cells) after prolonged use, thus permanently reducing the bone marrow reserves.

Low white blood cell counts are usually the most severe side effect of chemotherapy and in many cases limit the frequency of treatments. Low white blood cell counts make people much more susceptible to infection; people receiving chemotherapy should not be exposed to anyone with a cold or virus. If a person receiving chemotherapy develops a fever of any kind, they should be evaluated immediately by their physician. If their white blood cell count drops to very low levels, they may need to be hospitalized and given prophylactic (preventive) antibiotics. Recently, a medication has been developed using genetic engineering that can increase the body's production of white blood cells. While it can't prevent the reduction of white blood cell counts after chemotherapy entirely, it can minimize the severity of the problem.

Chemotherapy can also affect the red blood cells, leading to anemia. Although this is a common side effect of chemotherapy, it is usually not severe. Erythropoietin, a hormone that directs the body to manufacture more red blood cells, is now available as a medication that can help prevent anemia. Platelets, the small sub-cells in the blood that cause clots to form, are also reduced during chemotherapy. This can result in easy bruising, nosebleeds, or bleeding from the gums. If platelet counts become very low, a platelet transfusion may be required. This is quite rare, though.

Chemotherapy has several effects on the gastrointestinal system. Nausea and vomiting are thought to occur because the chemicals directly stimulate the vomiting center in the brain. The likelihood of suffering nausea and vomiting varies dramatically according to which chemotherapy agent is being used. Cisplatin and bleomycin almost always cause severe vomiting, for example, while methotrexate and fluorouracil rarely cause even mild nausea. When nausea does occur, it will usually begin between thirty minutes and three hours after the chemotherapy is administered and may last for a day or two. Several new medications have been developed within the last seven years that can effectively prevent, or at least minimize, nausea and vomiting during chemotherapy.

The direct effects of chemotherapy on the lining cells of the gastrointestinal system can also cause several effects. Ulcerations of the mouth, throat, and intestine occur in some cases but can usually be treated by simple mouthwashes and medications. Diarrhea may also occur, but again is easily treated in almost every case. Loss of appetite can be a symptom of the cancer itself, but may be made worse by chemotherapy. Food supplements and even medications that increase appetite can help minimize weight loss during this time.

Some chemotherapy drugs cause hair loss, of course, usually beginning about two weeks after the first treatment. In almost every case, hair growth returns once chemotherapy is completed. Some people's hair even seems to get used to chemotherapy. They will lose hair during the first few treatments, but their hair growth (rate) subsequently returns to normal well before treatments are complete.

Chemotherapy also interferes with reproductive functions, reducing sperm production in men and stopping egg maturation in women. These effects may or may not return to normal after the chemotherapy is complete. Patients who wish to have children can have eggs or sperm stored (frozen) before beginning chemotherapy.

A few chemotherapy drugs can damage the distant nerve endings in the hands and feet, causing numbness and tingling sensations. Although these side effects are usually temporary, it may take several months for normal sensation to return after chemotherapy is finished. One chemotherapy drug, cisplatin, can also damage the nerve endings in the ear resulting in hearing loss. People receiving cisplatin should undergo a hearing test every few weeks. If hearing loss begins, treatment can be changed to another drug before any serious loss occurs.

Finally, because chemotherapy drugs work by interfering with DNA, they may themselves be carcinogens (cause cancer). Long-term survivors of chemotherapy are at a higher risk of developing a second cancer than are people who have never had chemotherapy. An increased risk of acute leukemia has been reported within a few years after chemotherapy, while other tumors aren't likely to develop for decades. The risk of developing a second cancer is not huge, but rather is similar to that seen in people who smoke or have occupational exposures to carcinogens. In any case, the priority must be focused on curing the cancer a person currently has, not worrying about effects that may not be seen for twenty years or more.

Cortisone

Any treatment that damages or destroys cells can cause swelling. This is a greater problem with chemotherapy than radiation or surgery, since the effects of chemotherapy often involve the entire brain to some extent. Cortisone-type steroids such as dexamethasone (Decadron), prednisolone, and predinisone are usually given following chemotherapy to reduce this swelling. They may also be given on a long-term basis to control swelling caused by the tumor itself. Although these drugs are not really chemotherapy agents, they are included in most chemotherapy regimens for these reasons.

Cortisone has several side effects. During short-term use, many patients experience an alteration of mood (either euphoria or depression), difficulty sleeping, and fluid retention. People with diabetic tendencies will also experience elevation of blood sugar and may require increased amounts of insulin (or may need insulin for the first time). Cortisone can also cause easy bruising and menstrual irregularities.

When a person takes cortisone for a longer period of time, they may develop symptoms such as slow wound healing, thinning of the skin, stomach trouble (heartburn or even ulcers), and abnormal fat deposits in their face and across their upper back. At the same time, their body stops making its own cortisone, so when the drug is stopped it must be tapered slowly to allow the body time to adjust. With acute long-term cortisone use osteoporosis and fractures can develop, as well as cataracts, glaucoma, and generalized muscle wasting.

INTRATHECAL (IN THE SPINAL FLUID) CHEMOTHERAPY

When the best chemotherapy drug for a tumor is one that cannot cross the blood–brain barrier, it is necessary to administer chemotherapy directly into the cerebrospinal fluid. The most common means of doing this is by inserting a device called an Ommaya™ Reservoir. The reservoir is somewhat similar to a Port-a-Cath, except that the injection port is inserted under the skin of the scalp. Using local anesthesia, a small hole is drilled in the skull and a small tube passed from the injection reservoir into one of the ventricles of the brain. Chemotherapy can then be injected directly into the cerebrospinal fluid.

An alternative method is sometimes used when a craniotomy has been performed to remove most of the tumor. Small, absorbable wafers saturated with chemotherapy drugs are inserted into the cavity formed by the tumor's removal. They will slowly dissolve, releasing the chemotherapy drug into the area of the tumor.

At this time the only approved form of implantable chemotherapy is Gliadel® wafers, which release a chemotherapy drug called BCNU, the standard chemotherapy used to treat glioblastomas. Gliadel wafers deliver a high dose of BCNU to the tumor bed while very little of the drug reaches the rest of the body, thus minimizing side effects. Other forms of implantable chemotherapy would be available within a few years.

New Advances in Brain Tumor Treatment

Most of the advances currently being developed to treat brain tumors are used in addition to standard surgical, radiation, and chemotherapy treatments. I must emphasize that there is no single therapy on the horizon that holds promise of a cure for currently hopeless cases. The treatments discussed below show promise of prolonged survival and improved outcomes. But none offer a complete cure to those who would otherwise not survive.

In some cases, these newer therapies are available only to people participating in clinical studies of the treatment. While this may mean travelling to a study center to receive the treatment, it could certainly prove worthwhile for those with difficult to treat tumors. For that reason, a discussion of exactly what a clinical trial involves is placed at the end of this section.

Immunotherapy is any type of treatment that uses the body's immune system to help "reject" and kill tumor cells. The immune system provides some natural defense against cancer, attacking and killing cancer cells that do not carry the body's "markers" showing the cell to be a natural part of the body.

The immune system's activity is regulated by hormone-like chemicals called biological response modifiers, or BRMs. Immunotherapy uses BRMs manufactured through genetic engineering to either stimulate a person's immune system to fight the tumor, or in some cases kill the tumor directly. While most research in this area remains at the laboratory animal stage, several biological response modifiers now are in clinical use. Alpha interferon is an example of an immune therapy currently available for general use.

Viral therapy uses genetically modified viruses that attack and kill tumor cells without damaging the surrounding normal cells. Several modified viruses are in early investigation for brain tumor treatment, and one or more will probably enter clinical trials within two years.

Angiostatic therapy attacks the growth of new blood vessels that supply the tumor with nutrients and oxygen. Without an adequate blood supply, the tumor will not be able to grow. Phototherapy is one type of angiostatic therapy. During phototherapy, the patient is injected with a light-sensitive drug that is known to concentrate in a tumor, and then the tumor is surgically exposed and a laser light is focused on it. The light activates the drug, which then damages the blood vessels that supply the tumor.

Radiosensitizers are drugs that enable tumor cells to be killed easily using radiation. Taxol is a radiosensitizing drug used frequently prior to radiation therapy for brain tumors. Recent research suggests that some recurrent tumors that have always been considered resistant to radiation may be sensitized by taxol, making radiation effective. Other radiosensitizers are currently in development.

One of the most promising fields of research concerns the abnormal genes, known as oncogenes, that direct cancer cells to constantly divide. Proto-oncogenes are the normal genes that direct a cell's growth and development. If these become damaged or are genetically incorrect, they can become oncogenes, directing the cell to divide and grow constantly resulting in a tumor.

Oncogene research is beginning to determine what events cause a proto-oncogene to become an oncogene. As more is learned about the process, it is hoped that it will lead to ways to turn the oncogenes "off" so that they stop directing cancerous cells to divide.

CLINICAL TRIALS

A clinical trial is an organized study conducted to answer specific questions about a new treatment or new way of using a known treatment. Clinical trials may involve new anticancer drugs, new combinations of drugs being used, or new ways of administering a treatment. In most cases, clinical trials compare the best standard therapy with a newer therapy to see if one produces more cures and causes fewer side effects than the other.

Before a treatment is made available for clinical trial, it is studied carefully in laboratory animals. After that it is allowed to be used in carefully controlled clinical trails in people, proceeding through several phases of trial, each with its own rules and regulations. Phase I studies determine the safety and safe dosage range of a drug. This typically involves only a small number of patients, often studied one or two at a time. Small doses are given at first and then increased until side effects begin to develop. Phase I studies are generally offered only to cancer patients whose tumor cannot be helped by any known treatment. They do not determine if a treatment is effective or not— only if it is safe.

Phase II studies are designed to see if the treatment is actually effective. These studies involve more people (usually twenty-five to fifty, all having a specific type of cancer). Patients with tumors that are not responsive to standard therapies are eligible to participate in Phase II studies, but only a few centers will conduct the study. Because more people participate than in the Phase I study, some treatment of side effects may not become apparent until this phase of study. For Phase II studies of cancer treatments, the study is usually considered effective if 20 percent or more of the participants evidence shrinkage of their tumor. Phase II studies do not determine if the treatment is better than other treatments, only if it might prove effective.

Phase III studies compare a treatment that has been successful in Phase II trials to the accepted treatment for a certain type of cancer. Phase III studies are large, consisting of hundreds or even thousands of patients studied in a dozen or more different centers. Patients are randomized in a Phase III study; some receive the new drug while others receive the standard treatment. It is important to realize that participating in a Phase III study does not guarantee that the person will actually receive the study medication. Only after Phase III studies are complete will it be determined if the drug may prove better than the standard treatment.

Some treatments will enter a fourth phase, called Group C studies. These are usually drugs or treatments awaiting Food and Drug Administration (FDA) approval that are available to certain doctors or treatment centers (usually those who performed the Phase III studies) to continue to use and collect further data.

Participating in clinical trials is an individual decision. The advantages may mean access to drugs not yet available to the general public, and often free care and treatment during the course of the study. Participation could mean free follow-up care for years after the study is completed. On the other hand, there can be real risks involved. Some treatments that initially appear effective are later found to be not as good as the standard (existing) therapy, while others are found to have long-lasting side effects that weren't expected.

If you are interested in learning about which studies are available, the National Cancer Institute (NCI) has created a computer file about cancer clinical trials called Physicians' Data Query (PDQ). The information in PDQ is updated monthly with the latest information on clinical trials being offered around the country. Patients can obtain PDQ information by contacting the Cancer Information Service (see appendix C).

There are other studies that do not take place directly under the auspices of the FDA or NCI. These may include studies organized by medical schools or sponsored by manufacturers of certain drugs or products. In any case, legitimate research studies do not charge you or your insurance company if you participate. It is unfortunate, but there are health care providers who advertise so-called research treatments in order to attract patients that they can bill for their services. In almost all cases, the exact same service is available near your home.

Long-Term Outcome

Unfortunately, brain tumors are such a diverse and complex group of tumors that it is impossible to make generalizations about their long-term outcome. When a tumor is benign, the neurosurgeon will be able to tell you if it was completely resected during surgery, and therefore cured. Unlike malignant tumors in other parts of the body, however, surgeons often cannot tell if a malignant brain tumor was completely resected during surgery or not.

Usually a follow-up MRI scan will be obtained a few days after surgery once chemotherapy or radiation therapy has been completed, and again six months or so after all treatments are finished. Even then, it may be a year or more before the neurosurgeon is comfortable that you are cured and is of the opinion that the tumor is unlikely to recur.

In the meantime, there are superb support groups available for brain tumor patients and their families. Your doctor and hospital can often put you in touch with groups in your area, and a host of national organizations with regional chapters (several are listed in appendix C) are available.

The Internet has become a wonderful tool to both learn about your particular disease and contact others for support and information. It's important to always remember, however, that the Internet is not edited nor subject to review by professional organizations. A lot of people can launch very professional-looking Internet sites and state anything they please, which may or may not be based on facts.

PART IV

Other Neurologic Diseases

CHAPTER 14

Traumatic
Brain Injury

Traumatic brain injuries include any incident or trauma that caused physical damage to the brain. The severity of brain injury ranges from widespread destruction of brain tissue that causes death to very minor damage caused by a concussion (temporary unconsciousness). While everyone understands that someone with a gunshot wound to the head will suffer severe brain damage, most people do not realize that significant brain damage can occur in the absence of a skull fracture.

In the U.S., about 375,000 people suffer significant traumatic brain injury each year. Of these, 56,000 persons will die from the injury, and another 100,000 people will suffer lifelong disability. According to the National Brain Injury Foundation, the cost of traumatic brain injuries in the U.S., including lost production, wages, and long-term care, is estimated to be from $25 to $40 billion annually.

These statistics reflect only major brain injuries. As many as seven million minor head injuries are reported in the U.S. each year. More and more evidence shows that even people who suffer the most minor of brain injuries can have mental problems for months or years afterward.

Tragically, brain injuries are most likely to affect the young. More than 30,000 children sustain permanent brain injury each year, and over 70 percent of all brain injuries occur to persons under age thirty. Males are twice as likely to suffer brain injury as females, but the rate for females is increasing rapidly as more women become involved in contact sports and outdoor activities.

The primary cause of brain injury is motor vehicle accidents, which account for about half of all cases reported in the U.S. Falls are the second leading cause of brain injury, causing about 20 percent of all cases, followed by gunshot wounds (12 percent) and recreational and sports injuries (10 percent). Alcohol is an important contributing cause: Almost half of all people suffering traumatic brain injury were intoxicated at the time it occurred.

There is some good news, however. The death rate from traumatic brain injury decreased 20 percent between 1980 and 1992, due almost entirely to a dramatic drop in the number of people injured in motor vehicle accidents.

How the Brain Is Injured

Every brain injury is slightly different. Even two injuries that appear quite similar may have very different outcomes. However, the events that injure the brain are basically the same in every case. Generally, the mechanisms of brain injury are divided into primary events (which happen during the injury) and secondary events (those that happen hours or days later).

PRIMARY BRAIN INJURY

Primary injury involves the direct transfer of force to the brain. The brain is well protected from outside forces, being encased in the bones of the skull and floating in a bath of cerebrospinal fluid. The brain can still be injured in several ways during a traumatic event, however.

Lacerations (tears of the brain tissue) can occur anytime the skull is broken or pierced. Fragments of skull bone, or any foreign object that enters the skull, can tear through delicate brain tissue.

Even if the skull remains intact, the brain can be significantly injured. Cerebral contusions (bruises of the brain) can occur if the brain is bounced against the walls of the skull. A severe impact, such as a blow to the head or a fall, can cause the skull to move so quickly that it strikes the surface of the brain, which is floating inside. The brain stem, frontal lobes, and temporal lobes are most likely to suffer cerebral contusions because they are closest to the walls of the skull. In rare cases, this "bouncing" of the brain can cause a laceration of the brain tissue, even though the skull is not fractured.

When the brain bounces inside the skull, two areas are most likely to be bruised. The first injury affects the area of the brain directly under the blow. This is called a coup injury and occurs when the skull is driven directly back onto the brain's surface. The second injury occurs on the side of the brain opposite the coup injury. It is called a contrecoup and occurs when the brain bounces away from the first impact and hits against the opposite side of the skull.

A skull fracture or laceration can (obviously) break blood vessels within the skull causing a hematoma (blood clot) to develop. Even a severe contusion can tear delicate vessels within the brain tissue. Hematomas usually occur between the skull and the brain (epidural or subdural hematoma), but sometimes they are located deep within the brain itself (intracerebral hematoma). Small hematomas may resolve by themselves, but large ones must be removed surgically before the pressure they cause crushes brain tissue.

The most subtle form of primary brain injury is called a diffuse axonal injury. Diffuse axonal injury occurs when the brain stretches suddenly or rotates, resulting in a tearing injury to the long bundles of nerve fibers (axons) that travel from one part of the brain to another. Because there is no laceration or bleeding, diffuse axonal injury cannot be seen on a CT or MRI scan. Even when it is severe, the only abnormality noticed is a generalized swelling of brain tissue. In mild cases, only minor symptoms are caused by a diffuse axonal injury, and they clear up over a few weeks or months. In severe cases, coma and severe brain damage may result.

SECONDARY BRAIN INJURY

After the brain is injured, a series of chemical changes occur at the cellular level that can cause further damage. Recent research suggests that these changes actually destroy brain cells and connections between the cells that might otherwise recover. It has long been known that swelling around the injury can cause further damage, just as it does in persons who have suffered a stroke or who have a brain tumor. It is now known that injured brain cells also release several different chemicals and neurotransmitters (the chemical messengers between neurons) that can damage nearby cells.

Most recent studies suggest that damage to the brain's blood vessels is the major cause of this secondary brain injury. After injury, the brain's blood vessels lose their ability to regulate the amount of blood flow, and the blood–brain barrier doesn't function properly in the damaged area. This change occurs within six hours after injury, and can continue for up to six days. It is this change in the blood vessels that causes much of the swelling observed after a brain injury.

At the same time, the brain cells destroyed by the initial injury rupture, releasing their internal contents. Some of the chemicals released by the dead cells are toxic to surviving cells in the area, and may cause these other cells to die. The chemicals worsen swelling in the area and also worsen the abnormalities of the blood vessels and the blood–brain barrier. The problem is even worse if bleeding has occurred because iron and other products released by dying red blood cells are also toxic.

In summary, the actual brain damage caused by the initial injury may become much worse because of secondary biochemical events that occur after the injury. Although research is examining methods of preventing these biochemical changes, it is still not certain how they can be effectively prevented.

ANOXIC BRAIN INJURY

Anoxic simply means lack of oxygen. Anoxic brain injury can occur in any of several ways. Drowning or suffocation prevents oxygen from entering the body, while cardiac arrest prevents the blood from carrying oxygen to the tissues. In either case, the brain is the organ most likely to be damaged since its cells have the least ability to live without oxygen. When events such as these damage the brain, it results in diffuse (meaning widespread) anoxic injury. Diffuse anoxic injury usually occurs only in people who have suffered multiple injuries involving several parts of their body.

Even if breathing and heart function are normal after an injury, swelling in parts of the brain can be so severe that blood flow cannot reach the tissue in that area. This will cause a localized anoxic injury. A localized anoxic injury is not very different from a stroke.

What Are Concussion and Coma?

CONCUSSION

The two extremes of brain injury—with the exception of death—are concussion and coma. Concussion occurs when there has been a mild injury or bruise to the brain, and is commonly described as "getting your bell rung" or "seeing stars." The hallmark of concussion is a short loss of consciousness, or near loss of consciousness. Near loss of consciousness may mean a person is dizzy and can't stand up, or can't really focus on their surroundings even though they are awake. Concussion can be caused by any impact to the head or face, such as a fall or punch.

After regaining consciousness, most people will continue to exhibit signs of concussion for a few minutes to a few hours. These
symptoms include disorientation to time and place, difficulty with
coordination, a vacant stare, confusion, and headache. Many people
feel and look perfectly normal within a few minutes of regaining
consciousness.

In the vast majority of cases, a concussion causes no long-term
problems. Some people will continue to have a headache, mild dizziness, or trouble thinking clearly for a day or two. It isn't unusual to
have retrograde amnesia (an inability to remember things that happened just before the injury) or anterograde amnesia (an inability to
remember things that happened just after the injury). Complete amnesia—when a person doesn't know who they are or remember their
past—is incredibly rare in real life (although quite common on television daytime dramas). In the rare cases when it does occur, complete
amnesia is more often caused by psychological trauma rather than
physical injury.

A few people who have suffered a concussion continue to have
some long-term symptoms, however. This is usually called mild traumatic brain injury and is discussed in more detail below. Mild traumatic brain injury is much more likely to occur when a person suffers
a second concussion before the first is completely resolved. This is
called the second impact syndrome, and is believed to result because
healing from the initial injury is not complete, making the brain tissue susceptible to widespread damage from the second injury. It is because of the second impact syndrome that football players should not
be allowed to return to a game after suffering a mild concussion, even
if they feel perfectly normal.

Repeated concussions, such as those suffered by boxers, can cause
a progressive deterioration in brain function even if they did not occur
close together. This presumably occurs because each concussion
leaves a bit of damage behind, which, by itself, would not be significant but when added together results in many small areas of damage

throughout the brain. This was once referred to as being "punch drunk" because people typically have trouble balancing, have slurred speech, and are not able to think or remember things very well.

COMA

Most of us think of coma as a deep sleep from which a person can't be roused. Medically, the word *coma* simply means "unconsciousness." There are different degrees of unconsciousness that the word coma can refer to. With complete unconsciousness a person will not respond to any amount of stimulation, even pain. During lesser degrees of unconsciousness, a person may respond to noise or pain by withdrawing or making facial grimaces, or even by opening their eyes. On television a person in a coma often sits up one day and is all better. In reality, recovering from coma is a gradual process, often followed by a long rehabilitation.

A coma following brain injury does not necessarily mean a bad outcome. Most people will eventually emerge from the coma. Some of them will recover completely over time, while others will be left with significant disabilities. A few may remain only minimally conscious (sometimes called a vegetative state) for years.

There are a variety of ways for doctors to evaluate how severe a coma is. The Glasgow Coma Scale (Table 14.1) is used to determine the depth of a coma and to monitor whether a comatose patient is improving or getting worse. Low Glasgow Coma Scores, and worsening scores, suggest severe or ongoing damage. Patients with a Glasgow Coma Scale of less than eight have a 50 percent survival rate, and many of those who do survive will have long-term problems. Patients with scores greater than twelve almost always survive, and most do well. Electroencephalograms (EEGs) and evoked potentials are also used to monitor brain function in comatose patients.

Unfortunately, it is sometimes necessary to decide if a person is in a deep coma or is "brain dead," particularly if the possibility of organ

Table 14.1   Glasgow Coma Scale

Eye Opening	E
spontaneous	4
to speech	3
to pain	2
no response	1
Best Motor Response	**M**
Responds to Verbal Command	6
Responds to Painful Stimulus	
localizes pain	5
flexion-withdrawal	4
flexion-abnormal	3
extension	2
no response	1
Best Verbal Response	**V**
oriented and converses	5
disoriented and converses	4
inappropriate words	3
incomprehensible sounds	2
no response	1
E + M + V = _____	

Total score less than or equal to 8 at six hours after injury = 50% die
Total score 9 to 11 = moderately severe brain injury
Total score greater than or equal to 12 = minor brain injury

donation exists. It is important for family members to realize at this time that brain death is not a deep coma; it is an entirely different condition. Brain death means that almost all the brain cells have been destroyed and there is no chance of any recovery. During coma, most of the brain cells are intact but they are not functioning properly. Medically, the criteria for brain death include no electrical activity on the EEG and, in most cases, a study showing that there is a complete absence of blood flow to the brain. When no blood flow to the brain exists, there is no hope of recovery.

Determining the Severity of a Brain Injury

Once a brain injury has been diagnosed, family members are understandably anxious to know what degree of recovery the doctors expect. During the first few days after injury, always remember that "no news is good news." Most of the information the doctors will get during this early time will consist of new complications or worsening brain damage. Whenever they tell you "no change," consider this a good sign since during this time period many brain injuries worsen.

It is also important to remember that no two brain injuries are alike, and no two will have exactly the same outcome. Doctors are very uncomfortable in making long-term predictions after a head injury because they know only too well that the outcome is so unpredictable. All doctors have seen brain injury patients who were originally considered hopeless but recovered fully, and others who were initially thought to have only a minor brain injury but henceforth were never able to function normally.

There are a few measurements that can provide some general predictions about the severity of brain injury, however. Remember that these are only general predictions; there will be many exceptions who do better or worse than expected. The two most important observations made are how long a person was unconscious after injury, and how long the posttraumatic amnesia (unable to remember events happening after the injury) lasts.

The simplest classification uses these criteria along with any visible damage seen on an MRI or CT scan to divide head injuries into

Table 14.2   Classification of Brain Injury Severity

Mild   Loss of consciousness lasting fifteen minutes or less, posttraumatic amnesia lasting less than one hour. No apparent brain injury on MRI scan or CT scan.

Moderate   Loss of consciousness or coma lasting up to six hours, posttraumatic amnesia lasting up to twenty-four hours OR presence of a depressed skull fracture or apparent contusion (bruise) or localized swelling of brain tissue on MRI scan or CT scan.

Severe   Coma for six hours or more, posttraumatic amnesia of twenty-four hours or more OR any bleeding within the skull or generalized brain swelling on MRI scan or CT scan.

---

mild, moderate, or severe categories (Table 14.2). Using these criteria, it has been shown that patients with mild brain injury have less than a 1 percent risk of having long-term problems, while those with severe injury have more than a 20 percent risk of long-term problems. Obviously this simple score groups a lot of different injuries into the "moderate" category. There are other scales used to assess the severity of brain injury that try to make more accurate predictions, but none are widely accepted.

Consequences of Brain Injury

The long-term consequences of a brain injury can range from none at all to being in a vegetative state. Generally, the possible long-term problems a person may suffer following a brain injury are grouped into four categories:

1. Alterations of consciousness
2. Cognitive (thinking) difficulties
3. Physical difficulties
4. Emotional and behavioral difficulties

ALTERATIONS OF CONSCIOUSNESS

Mild degrees of altered consciousness, namely sleepiness and fatigue, are common for a few days after any head injury, including a simple concussion. Occasionally, these symptoms can continue for weeks and months. More dramatic alterations of consciousness—such as coma—occur when there is severe brain damage. Damage to certain parts of the brain stem and thalamus can also interfere with consciousness, even if most of the brain isn't damaged at all. These changes may improve over time, or they may be permanent.

COGNITIVE DIFFICULTIES

Cognitive difficulties affect a person's ability to think, learn, communicate, or remember. Cognitive problems include difficulty concentrating, slowed thinking, memory loss, impaired judgment, and many other problems. Depending upon the location and severity of their particular injuries, different people will have different problems. Often, one or two kinds of cognitive problems are readily apparent but other functions are completely normal.

Thinking and Memory Difficulty

Memory is the function most often impaired following brain injury. Memory problems are so common probably because memory requires several different areas of the brain to work together. Injury to any one of the brain structures involved in storing and retrieving information will interfere with memory. Usually, old memories remain intact, but the affected person will have problems remembering new information. Short-term (telephone number) memory is most often affected. In almost every case, memory problems worsen during periods of stress or confusion.

Difficulty concentrating is also very common after a head injury. Concentration problems are associated with damage to the frontal lobes, which are frequently injured in head trauma. These difficulties are usually worse when the person is tired, stressed, or attempting to perform several tasks at once. People with concentration difficulties are easily distracted and need a quiet environment to be able to think properly.

When memory and concentration are impaired, often there will be difficulty performing many everyday tasks. Keeping lists and having a rigid routine every day helps immensely, as does an environment free of distractions. Over time, most people find that their brain "relearns" how to remember and concentrate, and they can function more normally most of the time. When they are tired or stressed, however, their previous difficulties will often return.

Many people who have suffered a brain injury also feel that their thinking is slower than it once was. This is thought to be due to diffuse axonal damage, which has injured the connections between various areas of the brain. Again, the problem is usually worse during times of fatigue or stress and worsens due to distractions in the environment.

Language Skills

Although it is less common following injury than following a stroke (see chapter 7), some people will have difficulty with communication. This may be a dramatic and complete inability to understand or to form speech (called aphasia), but usually is not that severe. It may mean being unable to think of certain words that we should know, frequently using the wrong word when something else is meant, or having a difficult time understanding rapid speech. In any case, speech therapy can usually help to restore normal communication skills, although the process may take several months.

Impaired Executive Functions

Executive functions are subtle and complex types of thinking that we do every day. Making goals and long-term plans, understanding another person's point of view, summarizing a set of information, or realizing when something is an exception to a general rule are all executive functions. Some people who have suffered frontal lobe damage lose some ability to perform these executive functions, even though most other skills appear normal. Typically, the affected person doesn't realize anything is wrong, although others notice the change immediately. (Remember, being able to see things from another person's point of view is an executive function.)

In some cases, these functions will return to normal over time. In others, special psychological therapy using repeated exercises can help a person to restore these abilities.

Perceptual Difficulties

It is unusual for a brain injury to cause actual deafness or blindness, but problems processing information from the eyes and ears is not uncommon. For example, problems in judging spatial relationships can cause a person to bump into furniture that they see because they are unable to judge where the object is in relation to themselves. The ability to recognize something viewed from a different or unusual angle can be lost, as can the ability to recognize certain sounds. Perceptual problems are less likely to improve over time than are most other cognitive problems.

PHYSICAL DIFFICULTIES

Brain injury can, of course, lead to paralysis or weakness affecting a person's ability to move around and perform the normal tasks of daily living. It may also cause medical problems or complications requiring treatment. Common physical problems after a head injury include seizures, weakness or loss of coordination, muscle spasticity, reduced endurance, and pain.

Seizures

Seizures are caused by damaged cells or scar tissue within the brain. Any person who has suffered a brain injury is at some risk of developing a seizure disorder. People who have suffered a penetrating injury to the brain (bullet wound, depressed skull fracture, etc.) are at higher risk than those with blunt trauma. For those with blunt trauma, the risk is proportionate to the severity of brain injury (Table 14.3). The risk is also higher for people who are less than five years old or over age sixty-five at the time of their injury.

Seizures may begin within hours of the injury but may not first occur for over a year afterwards. In almost every case, the seizures can be controlled easily with medications once diagnosed. Usually doctors will try to stop the medications after a person has been seizure free for a year or more, but some people will require medications for the rest of their lives.

Weakness and Coordination Difficulties

Damage to the motor cortex, brain stem, and connecting pathways within the brain can cause weakness or even paralysis in one part of the body, similar to the paralysis that occurs after a stroke. Damage to the cerebellum and its connecting pathways can cause coordination and balance problems. Depending upon the exact damage, coordination problems can cause difficulty with skilled motor tasks such as typing, certain movements such as reaching for an object, or may cause walking and balancing problems.

Even a mild head injury can upset these functions; people often feel dizzy and uncoordinated for a day or so after a very mild concussion. As with recovery from a stroke, it may take months to relearn some of these skills after a severe head injury, and some may never return entirely.

When a brain injury results in paralysis or weakness, spasticity (rigid muscle contractions) may also occur. Whenever spasticity occurs, care must be taken to prevent contractures (permanent shortening of muscles). Stretching exercises provided by a physical therapist can dramatically lessen spasticity and also lessen the risk of contractures. Sometimes splints and braces are required to prevent contractures from forming.

Table 14.3   The Risk of Seizures After Brain Injury

Injury severity (see Table 14.1)	Seizure risk in initial 12 months	Seizure risk in 5 years
Mild	0.1%	0.6%
Moderate	0.7%	1.6%
Severe	7.1%	11.5%

Loss of Sensation

Almost any sensation can be altered after a brain injury: hearing, sight, touch, sense of smell, or even taste may be affected. Loss of touch sensations in part of the body can occur if the sensory part of the cerebral cortex is damaged. Damage to the occipital cortex can cause loss of vision even though the eyes are normal. Loss of the sense of smell is not uncommon whenever fractures of the upper face or front of the skull occur.

When sensory loss occurs because an area of the brain is bruised, a gradual return of sensation will probably occur over a few weeks and months. If the affected area was torn (which is usually noticeable on a CT or MRI scan) return of function is unlikely.

Fatigue and Headache

Most people who have suffered a head injury report that they become easily fatigued and that their other symptoms are worse when they are fatigued. This symptom will usually clear up slowly over time, but it is important that a person suffering from a head injury learns to prevent fatigue instead of trying to overcome it. Pushing too hard is a common source of frustration for head injury patients.

About one-fourth of people who suffer significant head injuries will have chronic headaches for at least two years after the accident. In some cases the headaches are caused by damage to muscles and bones near the base of the skull or damage to sinuses. In others, the cause is unclear. In any case, these types of headaches respond to the same treatments used for other chronic headaches: stress management, medications used to treat migraine headaches, and pain medications. The problem is common enough that it is discussed separately below.

Significant Brain Injury

INITIAL RECOVERY

During the initial hospitalization following a brain injury, management is very similar to that of a stroke patient. Persons with severe brain injury will usually stay in an intensive care unit for several days. Medications and perhaps mechanical ventilation (a breathing machine) may be necessary to reduce brain swelling and avoid any further brain damage. Medications may also be needed to treat seizures, muscle spasms, or to provide sedation if the patient is combative.

For the first few days, medical care focuses on preventing complications. Infections of the respiratory and urinary systems are common complications, especially if other injuries are present.

Respiratory problems may also require mechanical ventilation, especially if the patient can't swallow properly or if the chest has been injured. Whenever mechanical ventilation is required, the patient will usually need sedatives to prevent them from "fighting" the ventilator. A heavily sedated person will seem to be in a coma, but the nursing staff will always let you know that the condition is caused by either sedation or the brain injury.

If mechanical ventilation is required (or is expected to be required) for more than a few days, doctors may recommend performing a tracheostomy, the surgical insertion of a plastic tube through the neck into the windpipe. The tracheostomy is actually more comfortable for the patient than a breathing tube through the mouth or nose, and also avoids some of the complications those tubes can cause.

While a tracheostomy is in place, however, the patient won't be able to speak. Tracheostomy is not permanent. Once the patient recovers sufficiently, it can be removed and will heal with only a small scar.

Physical therapists will usually begin moving the patient's arms and legs within forty-eight hours to maintain muscle function and prevent blood clots from developing. If necessary, feedings may be given through a nasogastric tube (a small tube inserted through one nostril and into the stomach).

People in coma or with paralysis following a head injury are unable to turn themselves in bed and are at risk of developing bedsores. The nursing staff will change the patient's position in bed every few hours to prevent this from happening. They will also try to move the patient to a sitting position several times a day, if possible, because this helps prevent any long-term problems from developing. Sitting also helps prevent development of contractures and blood clots in the legs and may help lower pressure within the skull.

Once the patient has stabilized (usually four to ten days after a severe head injury), they will be transferred to a regular hospital floor. If necessary, they may then be transferred to a rehabilitation hospital for extended physical therapy before going home.

REHABILITATION

The healing process after a brain injury can last for months—or longer. Since the adult brain cannot make new nerve cells, any nerve cells that have been destroyed can never be replaced. As brain swelling decreases, many surviving brain cells will begin to function again. Damaged cells that survive can repair themselves and reestablish connections with other neurons.

Axons and dendrites (small fibers that connect nerve cells to each other) grow very slowly, however, and it can be months before the brain is fully "reconnected." Even after the connections are reestablished, the brain must "relearn" its new connections. The relearning process requires active rehabilitation. It has clearly been shown that those patients who undergo a rehabilitation program will function better, even years after the injury, than those who do not have rehabilitation.

Rehabilitation consists of two major goals: relearning and compensation. Relearning takes advantage of the fact that the brain is "plastic," that is, it has some ability to reorganize itself. Relearning allows the remaining nerve cells to take over some of the functions of the destroyed cells, and retrains brain cells that are healing after the injury. Several studies seem to indicate that relearning therapy actually helps speed the brain's healing. Relearning therapy is what we usually think of as physical therapy; therapists retrain patients to perform lost functions such as speaking or walking. It is a slow process, usually taking several months or more to complete.

Compensation therapy allows people to be able to function despite having permanent neurologic problems. For example, if a right-handed person has a paralyzed right arm, they can probably learn to write with their left hand. This (technically) is not relearning, since no part of the brain learns to control the right arm. Other compensations may involve using braces or assistive devices to help with physical skills, or learning techniques that will help a person to function close to normal despite lost mental skills.

The rehabilitation process after brain injury is different for each case. At first, particularly if the affected person has trouble with walking or self-care activities, the rehabilitation may take place in a rehabilitation hospital. The patient will spend several hours a day in a structured rehabilitation program of physical therapy and may have speech or other therapies as needed. As soon as patients are physically and mentally able to take care of themselves, they will be transferred to a day treatment program and return to living at home. Recovery usually progresses quickly during the first six months after injury, and then a bit slowly for the next two years. Improvement doesn't stop completely after two years, however. Many people, especially those who are under age thirty at the time of injury, continue to make slow but steady progress for several years.

People who have long-term alterations of consciousness, limited attention, or severe physical problems after injury may be transferred to a skilled nursing facility or nursing home. These facilities usually provide the same type of rehabilitation programs that a rehabilitation hospital does but at a lower intensity and for a longer period.

Many people with brain injuries require further treatment for specific problems long after they have returned home. This treatment may take place as outpatient therapy in a rehabilitation center but often can be provided by a home-health agency. These agencies can provide nursing care, physical therapy, speech therapy, and many other services through regular home visits. They are especially helpful for people living in rural areas who may have difficulty travelling to a rehabilitation center.

HOW THE FAMILY CAN HELP

As a patient recovers from brain injury, family members will begin spending more time with them. Once they have recovered consciousness, most patients will spend more time with their family members than with nurses and therapists. For this reason, it is important that family members know there are certain things they should and should not do around the patient. What is appropriate depends upon what stage of recovery the patient is in.

During coma, or whenever the patient is not responsive, it is important that family members realize that hearing is often the first sensation to return. Patients who have been in deep coma may later remember conversations that took place while they seemed completely unresponsive. Whenever you speak in front of the patient, assume that they understand what you are saying. Try to talk about positive things, speaking clearly and slowly. Focus on the patient, or speak about familiar people and things. If you like, you can assist the nurses and therapists by helping to give routine care such as shaving, washing hair, or helping to gently stretch and move the patient's arms and legs.

When the patient first begins to respond, the goal is to encourage even more response. It is important not to overload the patient with sensations, however. Patients will often become stressed by too much stimulation during this phase of recovery. Only one or two people should be in the room at any time, and there should never be several different stimulations taking place at once. For example, the television can be on, or a conversation may take place, but not both at the same time.

Similarly, when talking to the patient keep your response requests simple, one at a time, and do not continue them for too long. Asking the patient to squeeze your hand if he hears you is fine. Asking the patient to hold up two fingers, open his eyes, and move his legs will only cause confusion and frustration. Remember that the patient will usually become tired within ten to fifteen minutes at this stage.

As recovery progresses, confusion and agitation may become more apparent. Often the patient will not remember why he is in a hospital or what has happened. Because the patient's memory isn't working properly, he may ask the same question over and over. Again, be careful not to allow too many stimulations to occur at the same time. This will only worsen the patient's confusion and may cause more agitation. Respond in simple, calm tones and *do not* show that you are frustrated by having to answer the same question again and again. This will usually make the patient stop asking the question, but will leave him feeling very frustrated.

It may be helpful to provide visual clues to help the patient become oriented. A large calendar on the wall and a clock in an easily seen location are helpful. Try to keep a window shade open so the patient can tell if it is night or day (we can all become confused about that in a busy hospital). You may even post a schedule for meals and therapy sessions, or when certain people will visit.

As the patient continues to improve, it becomes important that family members let him take more responsibility for himself and become increasingly independent. During this stage, the patient may want to spend more time with other patients with whom he has developed friendships and less time with family. Often a parent, who has lived at the hospital—literally— for weeks, has a difficult time letting go at this stage. It is of paramount importance, however, that the patient learn to become independent again.

However, during the transition to home or assisted living, it does become important for family members to become more involved. Often, the home will have to be modified or equipment obtained to help with the transition. Some problems with thinking and memory that were not apparent in the hospital may become quite apparent once the patient moves to a home environment. Discuss the situation with the rehabilitation staff if you have questions.

Mild Traumatic Brain Injury (Postconcussion Syndrome)

Mild brain injuries (usually called a concussion) are far more common than the severe injuries discussed above. A mild injury (see Table 14.3 on page 237) is defined as an injury that causes loss of consciousness for less than fifteen minutes, with no accompanying structural damage severe enough to be seen on an MRI or CT scan. Millions of people in the U.S. suffer these injuries each year. Most of them return to normal within a few days or a week and have absolutely no other problems.

About 2 to 3 percent of people who suffer a concussion continue to have problems long after the injury, however. These people are said to suffer from mild traumatic brain injury, which is also known as postconcussion syndrome. Usually, the affected person was never even admitted to the hospital. They appear fairly normal, have no numbness or weakness, can walk and speak normally, and usually return to work or school expecting that everything will be fine.

The most common symptoms of postconcussion syndrome are chronic headaches, dizziness, difficulty concentrating, and difficulty with short-term memory. Alterations in mood including irritability, anxiety, and depression are also common. Most people also have some difficulty with the executive functions discussed on page 234.

Some people with postconcussion syndrome also have trouble with balance and coordination, although these are usually minor. Others feel that their thinking is slowed and that they have trouble focusing their attention, particularly if there are distractions present. Occasionally people have some minor difficulty with speech, such as being unable to remember a certain word. Others have trouble with planning or problem solving. The ability to draw, copy, and complete two- and three-dimensional constructions may also be affected as a result of mild traumatic brain injury. Impaired constructional ability can make even the simplest of home repairs quite difficult and may greatly interfere with the work of persons who operate machinery or perform assembly work.

The symptoms experienced by people with postconcussion syndrome vary from case to case; no person has all the possible symptoms. In many cases the symptoms occur only some of the time. Because the changes are subtle, people with postconcussion syndrome often find that others think they are just depressed, under too much stress, or are trying to make financial gains out of their injury. While these things certainly play a part in some cases, most people are sincere and are really experiencing problems.

Research has shown that all the symptoms of postconcussion syndrome can be caused by mild diffuse axonal injury, a stretching of the fibers linking one part of the brain to another (see page 227). These injuries have been found at autopsy examination of people who had postconcussion syndrome and have been re-created in simulation studies with animals. These injuries do not show up on a CT or MRI scan, and therefore can't be observed in a living person. Neuropsychological tests, however, can show the characteristic changes of postconcussion syndrome. These evaluations are the most sensitive method of detecting it and help decide what types of rehabilitation and treatment are most likely to benefit the affected person.

Neuropsychological tests (see also the section "Thinking and Memory" in this chapter) specifically evaluate the functions most likely to be affected by mild traumatic brain injury: verbal ability, memory, the ability to discern shapes and spacial relationships of objects, emotional function, vision, and hearing. The tests also evaluate problem-solving skills and executive functions and may also check hand-eye coordination, balance, and motor skills. While the major purpose of the tests is not to decide if someone has psychological problems, they can also detect how much depression or anxiety a person with brain injury is suffering from.

The tests results allow doctors and therapists to detect which functional skills are most impaired by the injury. This information can be used by physical and occupational therapists to set up therapy and retraining programs that can help restore lost abilities. With proper rehabilitation, more than two-thirds of people with mild traumatic brain injury can return to work and have complete return of their preinjury abilities. It is important that the problem be addressed early, however, as several studies have shown that rehabilitation takes longer if it is delayed for more than a few months after the injury.

Compared to therapy for major brain injury, rehabilitation following mild traumatic brain injury involves less effort in restoring motor skills and more effort on retraining thought processes. The therapy usually concentrates on problem solving, concentration, memory, and emotional or coping skills. Much of this is done through mental exercises, similar to going back to school for a few hours a day, but it is effective. Most people affected by postconcussion syndrome return to normal after having therapy for about three months. However, almost one-third will continue to experience some problems for at least several years.

Mild traumatic brain injury patients who have reduced productivity or on-the-job ability may benefit from the services of vocational rehabilitation counselors and occupational therapists. Their services may involve not only working with the patient to restore skills, but also working with the patient's employer to modify the job so that the patient can perform it without unnecessary stress.

People who have suffered mild traumatic brain injuries should be aware that the condition is considered a neurologic disability. This means that they are entitled to reasonable accommodations by their employer according to the Americans with Disabilities Act. Because the problems may not be readily apparent, however, it may be necessary to have a neuropsychologist clearly document them.

It may also be necessary for the person who suffers long-term symptoms to make lifestyle adjustments to cope with the problems. This may include structuring daily activities, making copious notes or recordings on audio cassettes, or structuring rest periods into their daily routine. Over time, many normal skills will be relearned and there will be a gradual return to a more normal lifestyle and level of function. Most people find that some activities will remain difficult for them for years after their injury, however, despite therapy and lifestyle changes.

Medications may help, at least in some cases. Antidepressant or antianxiety medications, along with psychological counseling, often prove quite helpful for those people suffering from depression, anxiety, or irritability. People who have difficulty concentrating may benefit from medication to increase alertness or help them sleep at night. Currently, some research studies are examining whether Aricept™, a medication developed for Alzheimer's disease, can help restore thinking abilities in people with mild traumatic brain injury.

As a final note, I should mention that there is sometimes confusion between postconcussion syndrome and an entirely different condition called posttraumatic stress disorder. Posttraumatic stress disorder is caused by severe psychological trauma, not by physical trauma to the brain. It can cause depression, anxiety, and sometimes difficulty with mental function, but is otherwise not similar to the effects caused by a mild brain injury.

CASE STUDY: Mild Traumatic Brain Injury

Sandra, a thirty-five-year-old saleswoman, tripped while walking down a flight of stairs and struck her head on the metal bannister. She was "knocked dizzy" as best she remembers. Bystanders helped her to her feet, but she felt very weak and had to lie back down for several minutes. Within fifteen minutes she was able to walk without help, although she still felt a bit dizzy. She declined suggestions to go to the hospital, since she already felt quite foolish and embarrassed.

When she got home she had a bruise on her forehead and a pounding headache. She used ice and Tylenol and went to bed. She had a bad headache the next day and left work early, but by the second day after her injury she felt better. She continued to have mild headaches almost every day, however. They weren't very severe and usually subsided with more Tylenol. She went to her doctor who found "nothing serious" and advised her that the symptoms would clear up in a week or two.

The headaches continued for several weeks, and Sandra noticed that she was having trouble concentrating at work. This was particularly troublesome since several times she found she had forgotten what a customer had just said. She also forgot an important lunch appointment. Although she was usually outgoing and quick-witted, she found herself struggling to maintain conversations. She also made several errors in judgment regarding sales, one of which led to a written reprimand by her boss.

She returned to her doctor who ordered an MRI scan of her brain, which was normal. He suspected she was under stress at work and gave her a few mild tranquilizers and sleeping pills. Sandra felt better on the medication, but her job performance seemed worse. She made several mistakes on order forms, missed another meeting, and her sales decreased steadily. Three months later, her boss gave her a final written warning, and she was placed on probation.

Sandra returned to her doctor, who asked a neuropsychologist to evaluate her. She spent an entire day in the neuropsychologist's office taking an exhaustive series of tests that determined that she had postconcussion syndrome with significant short-term memory problems. Sandra began a series of retraining exercise sessions with a therapist. At her doctor's suggestion, she transferred to a less stressful job in the firm. After six months, Sandra is still a bit forgetful, but finds that the adjustments she has made have allowed her to perform her new job without any problems. Her headaches have disappeared, and her friends say she's "her old self" again.

Specific Long-Term Problems Following Brain Injury

CHRONIC HEADACHE AND PAIN

Headache is the most common problem after a brain injury, reported by almost 80 percent of head injury sufferers for at least a few weeks. Interestingly, headache and other pain actually is more common after a simple concussion than after a major brain injury. The reason for this is not clearly understood. Chronic neck, shoulder, and back pain are also common, occurring in almost 50 percent of cases.

Doctors will usually order x-rays or other tests to insure that an injury to the neck or back was not missed during the initial evaluation, but these almost always prove normal. In most cases of neck and back pain, and some cases of headache, the pain is caused by muscle and tendon injuries and can be treated effectively by physical therapy. Even without treatment, most people report that their pain stops within six weeks after the injury.

Occasionally the pain persists for months, however. These chronic pain problems must be treated differently compared to any acute pain that occurs right after injury. If no obvious cause of pain is found, a chronic pain treatment center, which includes physicians and other health care providers from several different specialties, should be consulted. This can be quite important since chronic pain affects emotions, personal relationships, and can lead to physical dependence on medications if it is not treated carefully.

The headaches suffered after head injury are often called post-traumatic headache or postconcussion headache. These terms simply mean that the patient has a chronic headache following a head injury. The cause(s) of such headaches are poorly understood and are probably different in each case. In some people the headaches appear similar to vascular (migraine) headaches. Headaches may also be caused by muscles or other structures in the neck, and a few may be caused by irritation of the meninges (the linings of the brain) or pinched nerves. Typically, several of these problems contribute to the headaches an individual suffers.

Treatment of postconcussion headaches involves different therapies. When muscle spasms or pinched nerves are causing the headache, physical therapy or nerve blocks (injection of anesthetic around a nerve) can be helpful. If stress or tension are contributing to the headache then relaxation and stress management techniques can be of benefit.

Often, the treatment will also involve medication. Over-the-counter medications, such as Motrin® and Tylenol often help. Prescribed "pain pills" may be needed for severe headaches, but they should be used carefully. All these medications contain narcotics and will cause physical dependence if used every day for more than a few weeks. Additionally, whenever narcotics are used every day, they will quickly lose effectiveness and stronger medicines will be needed. This can result in a vicious spiral requiring more and more medicine to stop the headaches.

There are other types of medications that can be very effective to treat postconcussion headaches without the risks associated with pain pills, however. If the headaches have the characteristics of migraines, they may respond to migraine medications. Other medications, including certain antidepressants and antiseizure medications, can make the headaches less severe or less frequent. Most of these medications must be taken every day, rather than just when a headache occurs. Your doctor may have to try two or three of these medications before finding one that helps without causing side effects. The medications work slowly, so each medication trial may last several weeks. Overall, about 80 percent of people suffering postconcussion headaches report at least an 80 percent reduction in their headaches after treatment.

THINKING AND MEMORY

Thinking (doctors will refer to it as cognition or cognitive processes) is defined as "the mental process of knowing." Among other things, thinking includes sensing, memory, reasoning, and judgment. Obviously, thinking is a complicated process, and not surprisingly it can be affected by even a minor brain injury.

Memory itself (see chapter 3) involves linking information from several areas of the brain, storing the information, and then retrieving it as needed. We know that certain structures located deep inside the brain are active every time we try to remember something. Other specific parts of the brain are involved depending upon what we're trying to remember.

Problems with memory, especially short-term memory, are among the most frequent effects of brain injury. Memory difficulty may be the only symptom following a brain injury. Cognition (thinking) problems, on the other hand, rarely occur by themselves. Usually, a person who has cognition problems will also have memory problems.

When a brain injury victim experiences problems with thinking and memory, the only way to decide exactly which specific functions aren't working properly is through neuropsychological tests. Usually, the results of neuropsychological tests are divided into three broad categories called mentation, specific cognitive abilities, and executive functions. Each of these general categories includes several different types of thinking.

Mentation (which literally means "thinking") includes alertness, concentration, and mental stamina. Many people with a brain injury have difficulty concentrating, especially for long periods of time. Some also become easily distracted, or are unable to perform mental activities for very long without becoming fatigued. By knowing exactly which kind of problem the patient has, therapists can develop skills to help return their mental function to normal.

Specific cognitive abilities include knowledge and learned skills such as language, comprehension, motor skills, and visual-spatial skills. Many of these specific skills are processed in localized areas of the cerebral cortex (see chapters 2 and 3). Problems with specific skills generally develop only if there has been significant brain damage in those certain, specific areas. Some types of memory problems can also affect specific skills.

As discussed earlier, executive abilities include future planning, organization, control of impulses and instinctive drives, and self-awareness. Impaired executive functions often occur when there has been injury to the frontal lobes of the brain. They can also occur following minor traumatic brain injury.

People who have problems with any of their mental functions are understandably very frightened. Often they will deny there is a problem, though friends and relatives may be quite aware that something is wrong. The more severe the problem, the more likely the affected person will deny that anything is wrong. Often their fear is based on the premise that nothing can be done. In reality, mental functions can improve as much, or even more than, physical function after injury.

Thinking and memory problems are most severe just after the injury. They usually improve rapidly for the first six months after injury, and then improve slowly over several years. Individual people will recover differently, however. Some people will recover fully in a few months, especially if they undergo therapy. Others, especially young people with severe injuries, may continue to improve for years. It also isn't unusual for a person to appear to make little progress for several months, and then suddenly improve dramatically over the next month or two.

Mentation problems, such concentration difficulties, easy distractibility, or poor mental stamina, can be treated with medications. In other cases, they respond well to mental exercise and relearning techniques. Newer medications have recently been introduced that may help brain injury patients think more rapidly or clearly.

Problems with specific cognitive skills may require prolonged retraining. Because they may never return to complete function, learning ways to compensate for the problem may be the only available therapy. Problems with executive function are likely to slowly and steadily improve over time. Specific relearning and retraining programs in brain injury centers can dramatically help people whose executive functions are badly impaired. These are usually "live in" or all-day treatment programs that may last several months, however.

EMOTIONAL AND BEHAVIOR CHANGES

About one-third of people who suffer a significant brain injury will develop emotional or behavioral problems, especially if there was damage to the frontal or temporal lobes of the cerebral cortex. The most common emotional problems are depression and increased anxiety. A few people have episodes of sudden, severe emotion, such as weeping spells or rage attacks. These emotional outbursts may be started by actual events (weeping over a lost pencil, for example) or may occur suddenly for no reason at all.

Sometimes, the behavior problem is merely a symptom of poor emotional control. For example, a person may have consistent violent behavior when even slightly irritated. Other types of behavior problems, particularly involving changed sexual behavior, have no emotional component. These are apparently caused by damage to the specific brain centers that control social interactions.

Behavior problems can involve subtle things (inappropriate humor, inability to pick up another person's emotional clues) or may involve severe aggressive or destructive behavior, rage attacks, or inappropriate sexual behavior. In a few cases, people who have suffered a brain injury seem to have complete personality changes. In these rare situations, there is almost always destruction of a large part of the frontal or temporal lobes of the cortex.

No matter what its cause and no matter what form it takes, emotional and behavioral problems should be considered what they are: an inability of the brain to function normally. It's easy to be understanding when a loved one can't remember things or can't walk well following a brain injury. It's much more difficult to be understanding when he or she screams and yells for no reason.

It is also important to always remember that the injured brain is constantly relearning. If a person who suffers rage attacks gets whatever she wants every time she rages, she is getting positive reinforcement that rage works. If she gets to skip difficult physical therapy every time she has a weeping attack, she is getting reinforcement that weeping works (not to mention slowing down her physical recovery). It is important that family members, as much as possible, continue to behave appropriately even though the patient can't. Gentle insistence on appropriate behavior is the best method to retrain a person's brain to work properly.

Minor behavioral problems (yelling or emotional outbursts, for example) can usually be handled by the family at home. It is important that the family realizes they will have the largest role in correcting inappropriate behavior, since they interact with the patient more than anyone. The affected person requires consistent reinforcement from all family members. If reinforcement is inconsistent, the result is confusion and frustration for the patient.

Severe behavior problems that involve possible injury to the patient or others should be treated in an inpatient psychiatric or rehabilitation facility that has experience treating patients with brain injury. The treatment must be individualized for each problem, but in general consists of a behavior modification program that reinforces appropriate behavior and discourages inappropriate behaviors.

As with other types of brain injury, most emotional problems will improve rapidly over the first several months after injury, especially if the behaviors are not reinforced. In some cases, however, the problem becomes long term, particularly if it is not treated effectively during the rehabilitation process or if there was severe brain damage.

SPASTICITY

Spasticity refers to muscle spasms. In its milder form, it involves stiffened muscles in the arms and legs that cause movements to be jerky. In its severe form, muscles are so tightly spasmed that movement is not possible. Over time, the limbs can become frozen from these chronic contractions. Spasticity may also involve episodes of spasms—sudden, severe contractions of the muscles. Spasticity can interfere with rehabilitation to restore normal movements and also causes severe pain, especially during spasms.

The condition occurs whenever the brain sends abnormal signals to the muscles, telling the muscles to contract even though there is no reason for them to do so. Brain injury is only one of many causes of spasticity. It also occurs after strokes and spinal cord injury, and sometimes in chronic disease such as multiple sclerosis.

It usually isn't possible to stop spasticity completely, although some people will improve so much that the condition is barely noticeable. Physical therapy is effective in keeping affected muscles stretched sufficiently to prevent contractures (permanent shortening of muscles and tendons). Medications can also help to reduce muscle tightness and prevent spasms. In severe cases, surgeons may perform procedures that lengthen or cut tendons to avoid permanent contractures of joints.

Medications Used to Treat Brain Injury

The neurons (nerve cells) send messages to each other by releasing chemical transmitters called neurotransmitters (see chapter 1). The chemical is released at the connection between two neurons, allowing one cell to stimulate another. After a brain injury, some neurons may not release enough neurotransmitter, while other cells respond to neurotransmitters abnormally. Different cells in the brain use different neurotransmitters. More than two dozen different neurotransmitters have been identified at present, and more remain to be discovered.

Certain medications increase the production and release of certain neurotransmitters, while others drugs act as artificial transmitters, and still others can make cells more or less sensitive to some neurotransmitters. Although the brain is far too complex to allow us to pick a medication that works on one function (there is not a "vision" or "thinking" neurotransmitter, for example), there are circumstances where medications may help improve brain function after injury (Table 14.4, page 257).

Unlike choosing a specific antibiotic to treat an infection, a fair amount of educated guesswork is always involved in choosing the proper medication for certain neurologic symptoms. In most cases, the

doctor will know that a certain type of medication might help a particular symptom the patient has. It may be necessary to try two or three
medicines before finding one that helps the symptom without causing
side effects, or it may not be possible to find a medication that helps.

Two groups of medications commonly used after brain injury are
anticonvulsants (antiseizure medications) and antidepressants. Obviously, anticonvulsants are used when a person has seizures after a
brain injury, but they can also be effective in treating postconcussion
headaches and stabilizing sudden outbursts of emotion.

In addition to their primary purpose, certain antidepressants may
be used as sleeping pills, while others can be stimulants and improve
concentration. They are also used to treat postconcussion headaches
and chronic pain and may improve emotional stability. Some doctors
also believe that antidepressants reduce the frustration and irritability
some patients experience after brain injury. Both antidepressants and
anticonvulsants can be used for long periods without developing physical dependence on the medication.

Tranquilizers (Valium and similar drugs) are often used to treat irritability and anxiety following head injury. They are also the most effective drugs for treating spasticity and some types of muscle injury.
Some of these medications are also used as sleeping pills. All the tranquilizing drugs can worsen mental performance and increase confusion in some people after brain injury, however, and they may cause
physical dependence if used for a long period of time. Neuroleptics
(also called antipsychotics or major tranquilizers) are used in cases of
severe agitation and aggressive behavior.

Certain other drugs are used in rare cases, and should probably
only be prescribed by doctors specializing in head injury. Stimulants,
such as Ritalin® or amphetamines may improve concentration and
stop daytime drowsiness. Some of the newer drugs developed to treat
Parkinsonism and Alzheimer's disease *may* improve thinking ability
and mental endurance. (There is already far too much "hype" about
the potential of these medications, none of which have been studied

Table 14.4   Medications Used After Head Injury

Anticonvulsants
  Phenytoin (Dilantin®)
  Phenobarbital
  Valproic Acid (Depakote®)
  Carbamazepine (Tegretol®)
  Gabapentin (Neurontin®)
  Clonazepam (Klonopin®)
  Primidone (Mysoline®)
Antidepressants
  Amitriptyline (Elavil®)
  Nortriptyline (Pamelor®)
  Desipramine (Norpramine®)
  Fluoxetine (Prozac®)
  Clomipramine (Anafranil®)
  Sertraline (Zoloft®)
  Venlafaxine (Effexor®)
Neuroleptics
  Risperidone (Risperdal®)
  Haloperidol (Haldol®)
  Thioridazine (Mellaril®)
  Fluphenazine (Prolixin®)
Tranquilizers
  Buspirone (BuSpar®)
  Lorazepam (Ativan®)
  Diazepam (Valium®)
  Alprazolam (Xanax®)
Antispasm
  Baclofen (Lioresal®)
  Dantrolene (Dantrium®)

very thoroughly for this use.) Other medications may be effective against dizziness and help to control impulsive behavior.

Any medication—particularly those used to treat the brain—may cause side effects. In most cases, side effects such as sedation or dry mouth will clear up after a week or two on the medicine. If side effects are severe or don't clear up in a reasonable time, there are almost always alternative medicines that can be tried. In many cases, the medications are needed for a few months only while the brain heals.

CHAPTER 15

Meningitis and Infections of the Brain

At one time, infections of the brain (encephalitis) and the membranes covering the brain (meningitis) were among the most feared of all diseases, more lethal than most types of cancer are today, in fact. By the late 1950s, immunizations against viral infections had virtually eliminated some types of encephalitis, and antibiotics became available that could effectively treat most forms of meningitis. Some once-common causes of encephalitis, such as polio and mumps, were almost eliminated by the 1960s.

Unfortunately, other types of encephalitis and meningitis still occur regularly, often with devastating consequences. In fact, the frequency of these infections has increased steadily for the last decade, for several reasons. First, increased world travel has introduced new infections into areas that had previously never known them and where the population had no natural resistance against disease. The overuse of antibiotics has caused bacteria to develop resistance to the drugs (some bacteria are now resistant to virtually all antibiotics), making infections more difficult to treat. The HIV virus (Human Immune

Deficiency Virus—the cause of AIDS) not only makes its victims more susceptible to infections of the central nervous system, but the virus itself can infect the brain, causing encephalitis. Over one million people in the U.S. alone are currently HIV positive, and this group already accounts for a significant portion of all cases of encephalitis and meningitis that occur each year.

Bacteria and Viruses

If you are not clearly aware of the difference between bacteria and viruses, it is important to understand a bit about them before we discuss the different types of central nervous system infections. If you're already familiar with them, you may want to skip to the next section.

Bacteria are very small, single-cell organisms that can grow and reproduce almost anywhere that they can obtain food. Each bacteria contains most of the substances that the cells of our body contain: proteins, enzymes, DNA, etc. There are significant chemical differences between a bacterial cell and our cells, however. For example, bacteria have no nucleus, are surrounded by a thick membrane, and their enzymes are slightly different from animal or plant cells.

Antibiotics kill bacteria by interfering with one or more of these internal chemicals that differ from the chemicals in our cells. (For this reason, the antibiotic has absolutely no affect on us unless we have an allergic reaction.) An antibiotic may prevent the bacteria from dividing, or may prevent it from making new proteins, for example. Each antibiotic is effective against only certain types of bacteria—no single antibiotic can kill every type of bacteria.

When a physician treats someone with a bacterial infection, he must make two educated guesses: first, what type of bacteria is likely causing the infection; and second, what antibiotic is likely to prove effective against that bacteria. The educated guess isn't always correct, in which case the antibiotic does not stop the infection. When this occurs, the bacteria must be cultured (grown in the lab) and exposed to many different antibiotics. The doctor will then know exactly which antibiotics are effective against the bacteria and can prescribe the correct one. A culture usually takes about forty-eight hours to complete, however, which can be a critical amount of time during a severe infection.

Viruses are much smaller than bacteria (a normal bacteria can hold thousands of virus particles). Most viruses contain only the nucleic acid (DNA or RNA) that carries their genetic code and a protein covering. They cannot grow or reproduce by themselves because they don't contain all the working parts and enzymes of a cell. Instead, viruses must make their way into a "host" cell, where their DNA takes over the workings of the cell. Once viral DNA has taken over, it causes the host cell to stop its normal functions and instead make thousands of new virus particles. Eventually, the host cell bursts, releasing the new virus particles into the body (or out of the body to infect other people).

Because viruses don't contain enzymes and other cellular structures, antibiotics have absolutely no effect on them. (Yes, I realize that you get better when you take antibiotics for the flu, which is a virus. Sometimes this happens because you also have a bacterial infection. Usually, however, you get better after taking the antibiotics simply because people with the flu get better. Treating colds and flu with antibiotics is one of the major reasons bacteria are becoming resistant to antibiotics.)

There are some medications that can actually kill viruses, similar to the way antibiotics kill bacteria. Unfortunately, antiviral medicines are much more specific than antibiotics. Each antiviral medication works on only one, or at most a few, viruses. There are literally thousands of different types of viruses, and currently we have effective medications to treat only about a dozen. Antiviral medications are also more likely to have side effects and more difficult to use than antibiotics.

Meningitis

BACTERIAL MENINGITIS

Bacterial meningitis is an infection of the membranes lining the brain and spinal cord. It is by far the most common type of central nervous system infection. The typical early symptoms of bacterial meningitis are fever, headache, and a stiff neck. (Neck stiffness occurs because movement of the neck aggravates the irritated, swollen membranes around the spinal cord and brain stem.) Some people also have nausea, an abnormal mental state (usually feeling very sleepy, but sometimes even delirious), and a few will have seizures. When infants or the elderly have meningitis, however, these symptoms may not be present. The only signs of meningitis in these age groups may be irritability and a low-grade fever.

Frequently, meningitis begins as an infection of the sinuses, ear, or lungs that spreads to the meningeal membranes. In young children, the most common cause of this type of meningitis is a bacteria called Hemophilus influenzae (sometimes simply called H. flu). During the 1990s, a vaccine for H. flu became available, and it has markedly reduced the incidence of childhood meningitis. Strep pneumoniae, the bacteria that often causes pneumonia, is a frequent cause of this type of meningitis in older people. Many other bacteria can spread into the meningeal membranes from other parts of the body, however.

A few bacteria are capable of directly causing meningitis without any preceding illness. This type of meningitis often occurs during an outbreak or small epidemic. In older children and adults, these outbreaks are usually caused by a bacteria called Neisseria meningitidis. The outbreaks usually occur in crowded living conditions such as military barracks and college dormitories.

Bacterial meningitis is a medical emergency that must be treated quickly to avoid complications. For this reason, whenever a doctor even remotely suspects that a person may have meningitis, they will want to perform a spinal tap (see chapter 4) to obtain cerebrospinal fluid for analysis. Rapid tests on the fluid can confirm if meningitis is present with up to 95 percent accuracy. The fluid is also cultured to grow the bacteria causing the meningitis. If the doctor's first choice of antibiotics isn't working within forty-eight hours, the cultured bacteria can be tested to learn which antibiotic should be tried next.

In most cases of meningitis, doctors will want the patient admitted to the hospital to administer antibiotics intravenously (into a vein), since oral (by mouth) antibiotics do not work as rapidly. They will also want to monitor the patient to insure that no complications develop. Once definite improvement has been realized, which usually occurs anywhere from forty-eight to seventy-two hours, the antibiotics can be changed to an oral form and the patient is allowed to go home.

Before antibiotics were available, 90 percent of people who developed bacterial meningitis died. Even with antibiotics, as many as 10 percent of meningitis patients die, and others are left with permanent complications from the disease. Most of the complications are caused by inflammation and scarring of the central nervous system due to the infection. Complications are increasingly likely in very young children if there was a delay between the start of the disease and treatment or if the meningitis proved resistant to the first antibiotic used.

In young children, hearing loss (sometimes to the point of deafness) is the most common complication. Hearing loss occurs during the active infection, not after treatment. In infants, however, hearing loss may not be apparent at first and may only be noticed after the child has been released from the hospital. Administering cortisone early in the treatment of meningitis lessens the chance of hearing loss developing in infants and young children. Cortisone does not lower the risk of other complications developing, however, and is of no benefit in older children and adults.

Almost one-third of meningitis victims will experience at least one seizure. These may stop once the meningitis has been treated, but may continue long after the infection is over. In the latter case, the seizures are thought to result from scar tissue that remains once the infection has resolved. These seizures may be permanent but almost always respond well to medications.

Less frequent complications of meningitis include hydrocephalus because the infection interferes with the normal flow or reabsorption of cerebrospinal fluid. If this happens, it will be necessary for surgeons to place a shunt (see chapter 12) to drain the excess fluid to prevent brain damage. Other complications that occur but rarely include partial paralysis, loss of sensation in some part of the body, and loss of other functions caused by brain damage.

CHRONIC MENINGITIS

Certain forms of meningitis begin slowly, first with a mild headache, low-grade fever, and perhaps a stiff neck. Over days or weeks the affected person becomes increasingly ill and begins to experience all the symptoms of meningitis. They may also begin to have neurological symptoms involving the cranial nerves such as double vision, drooping of facial muscles, or loss of sensation (see chapter 1). Usually an analysis of spinal fluid will show all the signs of meningitis, but no bacteria will be grown when the fluid is cultured. The disease does not respond to the usual antibiotic treatments.

Most of these people will be found to have chronic meningitis—a type of meningitis caused by any one of several different organisms, all of which grow and reproduce much more slowly than the usual bacteria. Certain unusual bacteria can cause chronic meningitis, in particular the bacteria that cause tuberculosis, syphilis, and Lyme disease. Infections caused by fungus or yeast-like organisms can also cause chronic meningitis, as can a few other, rare organisms.

Doctors can usually determine that a person has chronic meningitis soon after admission to the hospital. It can be quite difficult and time consuming to determine exactly what organism is causing the infection, however. Blood tests may show if a person has tuberculosis or a fungal infection in a day or two, but actually culturing these slow-growing organisms from the cerebrospinal fluid can take several weeks.

Because tuberculosis is the most common cause of chronic meningitis, doctors may start treatment for tuberculosis until laboratory tests reveal exactly which organism is present. Tuberculosis treatment usually requires taking several different drugs for up to one year or more. Treatment of infections caused by spirochetes—the type of organisms that cause syphilis and Lyme disease—is simpler and more successful. Penicillin or another standard antibiotic taken for several weeks will usually clear up these infections. Fungal infections are the most difficult type of chronic meningitis to treat. The medications required must usually be given intravenously and are more likely to have side effects.

Even with rapid diagnosis and treatment, chronic meningitis has a high mortality rate and is likely to cause long-term complications. Spirochete infections can be treated effectively using antibiotics, and their outcome is similar to that of standard bacterial meningitis. Tuberculous meningitis is more difficult to treat, especially if it is caused by a strain of tuberculosis that is resistant to antibiotics. Fungal meningitis is the most serious type of chronic meningitis. Depending upon exactly which fungus has caused the infection, between 20 and 50 percent of patients with fungal meningitis will die.

All types of chronic meningitis are more likely to cause long-term problems than bacterial meningitis. Permanent nerve damage, seizures, and hydrocephalus all occur with increased frequency in victims of chronic meningitis, especially if a fungal infection is involved.

Chronic meningitis is much less common than bacterial meningitis because the immune system of most people can destroy these organisms long before they can develop into meningitis infection. Whenever a person develops chronic meningitis, doctors will carefully check their immune system to make certain that it is working properly. Chronic meningitis is much more likely to occur in people with AIDS, those taking anticancer drugs or cortisone for a long time, and people who have genetic problems with their immune system.

ASEPTIC (VIRAL) MENINGITIS

Some people who develop all the signs and symptoms of meningitis are found to have no bacteria or other organisms growing in their cerebrospinal fluid. These people are said to have aseptic (meaning "no infection") meningitis. Aseptic meningitis is usually caused by a viral infection, so it is often referred to as viral meningitis. A few other cases are caused by organisms called rickettsia and chlamydia, which are similar to bacteria. Occasionally, aseptic meningitis isn't caused by infection at all but is simply an inflammation of the meningeal membranes, usually the result of an allergic reaction.

Viral meningitis often occurs during outbreaks, usually in late summer or late winter. Certain viruses can cause meningitis year-round, however. In any case, most people with viral meningitis have the symptoms of a cold or gastrointestinal virus a few days before they develop meningitis. Some may only have noticed a low-grade fever and mild muscle aches. Frequently, doctors never determine exactly which virus is responsible.

In the vast majority of cases viral meningitis is not a very serious illness, although it can be a little scary. Simply treating the patient with rest and a mild pain medicine or anti-inflammatory drug, such as Motrin, will allow the disease to run its course in one to three weeks. There are rarely any long-term consequences after a routine case of viral meningitis.

A very few cases of viral meningitis can prove quite severe, however. People with severe cases usually have a high fever, very stiff neck, and altered level of consciousness. They may require hospitalization and treatment with antiviral drugs or cortisone. Even severe viral meningitis rarely causes hydrocephalus or hearing loss, but will sometimes result in seizures or mild brain damage.

Encephalitis

Unlike meningitis, which usually infects only the membranes around the brain, encephalitis always involves infection of the brain tissue itself. All cases of encephalitis are caused by viruses; bacteria and other organisms are not involved. Because viruses reproduce by taking over and eventually destroying brain cells, encephalitis almost always results in some amount of brain damage, although it may be so minor that it does not cause long-term problems.

The first symptoms of encephalitis are usually fever, headache, and fatigue. Extreme irritability, personality changes, and nausea may also be present. Within a day or two consciousness is impaired and the person becomes difficult to arouse. Some signs of brain damage such as a seizure, weakness, paralysis, or speech problems are usually apparent within the first three days of illness.

In the first half of this century, encephalitis outbreaks were caused by polio, mumps, measles, and rabies. Polio, mumps, and measles encephalitis were spread from person to person, and usually occurred in winter. Rabies encephalitis—spread by animal bites—was (and is) most likely to occur in the fall. Vaccination programs have dramatically reduced the number of encephalitis cases caused by these viruses, but a few are still reported each year, usually to people who were not properly vaccinated.

Today, herpes simplex virus is the most common cause of encephalitis, accounting for 10 percent of all cases occurring in the U.S. each year. Herpes simplex encephalitis tends to occur sporadically, rarely causing epidemics or outbreaks.

The other common forms of encephalitis are all caused by arboviruses, that is, viruses that are spread by mosquitos and biting insects. Because these viruses are spread by insects, they often occur in outbreaks or epidemics, usually in mid- to late summer. In the U.S., the most common causes of epidemic encephalitis are western and eastern equine encephalitis, St. Louis encephalitis, and Venezuelan equine encephalitis. In Asia and the Far East, Japanese B encephalitis is the most common cause of epidemic encephalitis.

Doctors can usually diagnose encephalitis by its clinical symptoms and via analysis of the patient's cerebrospinal fluid. An MRI scan will usually show inflammation and swelling in parts of the brain. It can take weeks to determine exactly which virus is causing the encephalitis. However, an educated guess can be made based on geographic location, the time of year, and what parts of the brain are most affected (different viruses have a preference for different parts of the brain).

Currently, only herpes simplex encephalitis can be treated with antiviral medications. Several antiviral drugs, particularly acyclovir, can destroy and prevent reproduction of the herpes virus. The only common side effect of the medication is interference with kidney function in a few people, but when this does occur, it is usually not severe. Herpes encephalitis had a 70 percent mortality rate before acyclovir became available; since that time its mortality rate is less than 20 percent.

For all other forms of encephalitis, the only treatment available is supportive care of the patient while their immune system battles the virus. The outcome depends on which virus is causing the encephalitis. Rabies encephalitis is always fatal, while eastern equine and Japanese B encephalitis are both fatal in about 70 percent of cases. Western equine encephalitis, St. Louis encephalitis, and Venezuelan encephalitis are rarely fatal.

Most people surviving either Japanese B or eastern equine encephalitis will have permanent brain damage. About one-third of herpes simplex encephalitis survivors will also have brain damage, while only a few people will have any serious effects after Venezuelan encephalitis. The most common long-term effects are mild difficulty with thinking and memory, personality changes, epilepsy (seizures), or permanent weakness or numbness in part of the body. Herpes simplex encephalitis is often associated with personality changes because it tends to infect the frontal and temporal lobes more so than other parts of the brain.

Postinfectious Encephalomyelitis

Postinfectious encephalomyelitis is a rare disease that is sometimes confused with encephalitis. The disease begins as a routine viral illness (most commonly influenza in the U.S., and measles elsewhere in the world) that appears to run its course. Days or weeks after the illness has ended, the person develops a low-grade fever and becomes very tired and weak.

Soon afterward they develop some sign of a problem in the brain: seizures, decreased consciousness, or loss of muscle function. When evaluated by a physician, their cerebrospinal fluid is usually normal. If a CT scan is performed, it will also be normal. An MRI scan, however, will show that some areas of the brain or spinal cord are inflamed and damaged.

The disease is actually an autoimmune reaction; the patient's immune system, which has recently been fighting a virus, has begun attacking the myelin sheaths that insulate the various nerve fibers. Because the reaction destroys the myelin, it is often referred to as a demyelinating disease, similar to the reaction that occurs in multiple sclerosis (see chapter 18). Researchers assume that an antibody the immune system made to attack virus protein can also attack some protein on the surface of myelin. Once the virus has been destroyed, these antibodies begin to attack the protein as if it were part of the virus.

Some centers treat this condition with cortisone or other medications to suppress the immune system, but this treatment has not been shown to be very effective. In most centers, the treatment protocol consists simply of supporting the patient until their immune system returns to normal and the brain heals. The condition is severe, however, and many people will require intensive care for several weeks before recovery begins. There may also be long-term damage, which will require rehabilitation.

Abscesses of the Central Nervous System

An abscess is an infection that collects into one space. When a bacterial infection enters the brain, the bacteria begins growing between the cells. As the body's white blood cells enter the area to begin fighting the infection, other cells begin to secrete connective tissue to "wall off" the infected area so that the bacteria can't spread to other parts of the brain. Eventually, the area becomes an abscess—a walled-off collection of bacteria and white blood cells commonly called "pus."

A pimple, for example, is a small abscess in the skin. Because the skin is made of very dense tissue and is close to the surface, however, a pimple will drain through the skin's surface before it gets to be very large or causes any real problems. Because the brain is made of very soft, loosely connected tissue and is located within the deep within the skull, an abscess can't drain through to the surface and can get very large.

The bacteria that cause an abscess usually reach the brain from an infection in a nearby structure. Chronic ear or sinus infections can spread to the brain, for example, causing an abscess in the frontal lobe or the brain stem, respectively. Bacteria from abscessed teeth, particularly the upper molars, can also spread to the brain. In some cases, the infection reaches the brain via the bloodstream. Pneumonia, an abscess in another part of the body (particularly the face), and any other infection that reaches the bloodstream can cause a brain abscess, though this rarely happens.

The symptoms of a brain abscess vary depending upon where in the brain the abscess is located. Most patients will have a fever and many will have headaches. As the abscess enlarges, symptoms develop due to the abscess's mass pushing against normal brain tissue. A brain stem abscess, for example, may cause weakness in the face and body or coordination problems. An abscess near one of the cerebral hemispheres can cause weakness on the opposite side of the body.

If the abscess continues to enlarge, then symptoms of increased intracranial pressure will develop, including vomiting, blurred, or double vision. Seizures may occur or the patient may experience symptoms similar to a stroke.

When a cerebral (brain) abscess is suspected, the final diagnosis is usually made by a CT or MRI scan that shows a fluid-filled cavity in the brain. A lumbar puncture to obtain cerebrospinal fluid usually doesn't aid in diagnosis because the abscess wall prevents cerebrospinal fluid from coming in contact with the infection. In fact, a lumbar puncture should not be performed if any symptoms of increased intracranial pressure are present since removing cerebrospinal fluid in such cases can worsen the patient's condition.

Treatment of an abscess varies according to its location. Because antibiotics have difficulty penetrating across an abscess wall, they are generally not very effective until the abscess has been drained. Surgery, usually involving a craniotomy (removal of part of the skull; see chapter 12), will be required to drain the abscess. In some cases, stereotactic surgery (see chapter 12) may be able to drain enough of the abscess so that antibiotics can work effectively. After the abscess is drained, several antibiotics are given in combination to treat the infection and insure that the abscess doesn't return.

Before CT and MRI scans were available, about 50 percent of people with a brain abscess died. Today, less than 5 percent of people with a brain abscess die, and more than half of the survivors have absolutely zero neurologic problems after recovery. Of those who do have neurologic problems after recovery, only 10 percent have such severe problems that they are considered disabled.

AIDS and Brain Infection

Although most people are familiar with HIV (Human Immune Deficiency Virus) and AIDS (Acquired Immune Deficiency Syndrome), many people are not aware of its effects on the brain. Between 50 and 70 percent of AIDS victims will develop neurologic complications from their illness. AIDS causes neurological problems in three different ways:

1. The HIV virus itself can infect and destroy brain cells
2. Persons with AIDS are likely to suffer other infections involving the brain
3. Some AIDS treatments can damage the brain. Often, AIDS victims will have several different neurologic complications during the course of their disease.

The HIV virus enters brain cells as well as white blood cells. Over time, it can destroy enough brain cells to cause major neurologic problems, eventually resulting in dementia (severely impaired thinking and memory). This syndrome, called AIDS dementia complex, is usually not present until the middle to late stages of AIDS. It usually begins slowly with symptoms similar to depression. As it progresses, memory loss, slowed thinking, and slow movements become apparent. Eventually speech is affected, and the complex may progress to the point that patients are mute and bedridden.

The changes in the brain that occur during AIDS dementia complex can be observed on a CT or MRI scan, although they may not be apparent until the complex has become severe. There is atrophy (shrinking) throughout most areas of the brain caused by the destruction of brain cells. Occasionally there are also plaques in the brain's white matter similar to those observed in multiple sclerosis (see chapter 18). These are especially likely to involve the brain stem where they will cause widespread effects. High doses of the medication Zidovudine (ZDV) can halt or slow the progression of AIDS dementia complex—at least for a while.

AIDS infection can also cause damage to the spinal cord and peripheral nerves. AIDS myelopathy is a condition resulting from damage to the spinal cord that occurs in some AIDS sufferers during the late stages of their disease. The condition causes severe weakness and loss of sensation in the legs but does not affect the arms and hands. Another condition, called digital sensory neuropathy, can also occur during the disease's late stages. The condition causes loss of sensation and severe pain, especially in the feet.

While the direct effects of the HIV virus on the nervous system can be crippling during the late stages of AIDS, infections of the brain caused by a defective immune system are a more common problem. In fact, a neurologic infection is the first symptom of AIDS in almost 10 percent of cases. Because of the abnormalities in their immune system, AIDS sufferers do not have all the signs and symptoms of a brain infection that would occur in other people. Additionally, they often suffer from infections by organisms that rarely infect other people.

AIDS patients may have viral or bacterial meningitis, but they are much more likely than others to develop chronic meningitis. Tuberculosis and two fungal infections, cryptococcus and coccidioides, are frequent causes of meningitis in AIDS patients. All these infections can be treated effectively with medications. Unlike other people, however, AIDS patients usually must continue to take a preventive dose of medication long after the infection has cleared. Without this preventive medication, they are very likely to have a recurrence of the meningitis.

Encephalitis is also common in AIDS patients. Herpes encephalitis is the most common type, although cytomegalovirus (a cousin of the herpes virus) is also a frequent cause. Antiviral medications are effective against both.

The most common cause of nervous system infection in AIDS patients, however, is an organism called toxoplasmosis. Toxoplasmosis rarely causes disease in people who have a normal immune system. In AIDS victims, however, it can cause pneumonia, cerebral abscess, meningitis, and encephalitis. Toxoplasmosis is more likely to cause a cerebral abscess than meningitis or encephalitis. Usually the patient's symptoms include headache and confusion. There may also be fever and stiff neck, seizures, or stroke-like symptoms.

A CT or MRI scan of a patient with toxoplasmosis will usually reveal several different abscesses. The only way to diagnose toxoplasmosis in an AIDS patient with certainty is by brain biopsy. Generally, treatment with antibiotics is effective, however, so most doctors will simply begin the medications. If the patient has not improved within a week or two, biopsy will then be required. Despite the frequency and severity of central nervous system infections in AIDS patients, they can usually be treated effectively and are rarely a cause of death.

CHAPTER 16

Alzheimer's Disease and Dementia

What Is Dementia?

Dementia is a term used to describe a loss of thinking ability, memory, or other intellectual capability that is so severe the affected person cannot function in everyday life. Dementia is not a disease, rather it is a set of symptoms that can be caused by many different diseases and conditions.

When it occurs in old age, dementia is often called senility. Even in old age dementia is not normal, however. Some slowing of mental processes inevitably occurs as we age, but many people continue to have good mental function well into their ninth decade and beyond. Dementia, even when we think of it as senility, is always caused by some underlying neurologic problem. Almost any disease that destroys a large part of the brain, or that interferes with general brain function, can cause dementia. For example, multiple strokes, a traumatic brain injury, or even severe depression can all result in dementia.

Table 16.1   Diseases That Cause Dementia

Neurodegenerative Diseases
 Diffuse Lewy body disease
 Parkinson's disease
 Progressive supranuclear palsy
 Frontotemporal dementia
 Pick's disease
 Olivopontocerebellar atrophy
 Progressive hemiatrophy
 Huntington's disease
 Amyotrophic lateral sclerosis (Lou Gehrig's disease)
 Postencephalitic Parkinsonism
 Prion diseases
 Multiple sclerosis

Other Neurologic Diseases or Injuries
 Brain tumor
 Hydrocephalus
 Chronic subdural hematoma
 Multiple cerebral infarcts (strokes)

Systemic (Involving the Entire Body) Diseases
 Vitamin deficiency (vitamin B_{12}, folate)
 Metabolic diseases involving thyroid, liver, or parathyroid glands
 Alcoholism

Infectious Diseases
 AIDS
 Neurosyphilis
 Encephalitis
 Meningitis

Psychiatric Diseases
 Depression
 Schizophrenia
 Manic-depressive illness (bipolar disorder)
 Severe anxiety
 Obsessive-compulsive disorder

There are also several neurologic diseases for which dementia is the major symptom. These are called neurodegenerative disorders, which simply means degeneration of the nervous system. Alzheimer's disease is by far the most common neurodegenerative disorder but there are many others (see Table 16.1, and the last section of this chapter).

What Is Alzheimer's Disease and Who Is Affected?

Alzheimer's disease was first described by Dr. Alois Alzheimer in 1906 when he performed an autopsy examination on a woman who had suffered severe dementia before death. When examining her brain tissue under a microscope, he noticed abnormal clumps and tangles of fibers where neurons (brain cells) should have been. He later examined the brains of other people with dementia and found the same clumps and tangles.

Alzheimer's disease begins quite gradually. The first noticeable symptom is usually forgetfulness about recent events. The disease progresses steadily until it causes confusion, behavior changes, and impaired thinking. Eventually, a person with Alzheimer's may be unable to complete a sentence or follow the simplest directions.

The disease affects different people in different ways, making it difficult to predict how an individual's disease will progress. Some people have severe symptoms within a few years, while others continue to function to some degree for up to twenty years. Even the specific symptoms vary from case to case. Some affected people will have severe emotional problems, while others are quite disoriented and can't think properly, while still others simply have memory problems.

Alzheimer's disease is the most common cause of dementia, affecting over four million Americans. Ten percent of persons over age sixty-five have Alzheimer's disease, while nearly half of those over age eighty-five have the condition. Because the average age of the population is increasing (as baby boomers age), it is expected that fourteen million Americans will have Alzheimer's disease by the year 2040.

There is also an early form of Alzheimer's disease that affects persons under age sixty (sometimes as early as their forties). This type of Alzheimer's accounts for less than 10 percent of cases, however. Most evidence suggests this early onset form of Alzheimer's is a slightly different disease than the more common form. Early onset Alzheimer's disease apparently is also genetically inherited to some degree since it occurs frequently in certain families.

Economically and emotionally, Alzheimer's disease is devastating. Currently, the average lifetime cost for each patient diagnosed with Alzheimer's is about $175,000. Alzheimer's patients fill approximately half of all nursing home beds (the average cost of nursing home care is $42,000 per year), even though 70 percent of Alzheimer's patients are cared for at home. Currently the total U.S. expenditure for Alzheimer's disease is about $100 billion per year, making it the third most expensive disease behind heart disease and cancer. The federal government spent about $350 million for Alzheimer's disease research in 1998.

Symptoms of Alzheimer's Disease

Alzheimer's disease begins slowly, usually with mild forgetfulness that can be explained away. As the disease progresses, it may become obvious that this forgetfulness is really symptomatic of a severe memory problem. During the disease's early stages, many people try to hide their memory problems by learning to cope using lists and written notes.

The Alzheimer's Association has developed a list of the most common early symptoms of Alzheimer's disease:

1. Memory loss that affects job skills. This may take the form of

frequent forgetfulness or unexplainable confusion at home or in the workplace.

2. Difficulty performing familiar tasks. Anyone might leave something on the stove too long or forget to serve part of a meal. People with Alzheimer's might forget they've even prepared a meal.

3. Problems with language. A person with Alzheimer's disease may forget simple words or substitute inappropriate words, which makes their speech seem garbled.

4. Disorientation to time and place. People with Alzheimer's disease may not know where they are, how they got there, or how to get back home.

5. Poor judgment, particularly in areas that have never been a problem. They may become targets for con men or scam artists.

6. Problems with abstract thinking. Performing basic mathematical calculations, such as balancing the checkbook, for example, may become impossible.

7. Misplacing things. In particular, a person with Alzheimer's disease may put items in inappropriate places—such as an iron in the freezer, or a wristwatch in the sugar bowl—and then not recall how they got there.

8. Changes in mood or behavior. Rapid mood swings for no apparent reason are common, as are nervousness and depression.

9. Changes in personality. Dramatic personality changes are unusual but sometimes do occur. Someone who is generally easygoing may become angry, suspicious, or fearful.

10. Loss of initiative. The person with Alzheimer's disease may remain disinterested and uninvolved in many or all of their usual hobbies.

Most people with early Alzheimer's will not exhibit every one of the above symptoms, but anyone who exhibits several of them should be evaluated by their physician. It is also important to remember that most of these symptoms can also be caused by depression, which is quite common in older people and easily treatable.

As the disease progresses, family members and friends will no longer wonder if there is a problem. The affected person may not recall conversations from yesterday and may frequently appear confused. They may have sudden lapses of memory that appear bizarre, such as forgetting they have just made dinner or being unable to remember how to get home from a friend's house.

Because of memory loss, a person with Alzheimer's disease often has an inability to learn new information. They may also repeat themselves or have difficulty carrying on a conversation because they forget the topic. Speech may become halting as the person struggles to find the right word. Balancing a checkbook or making judgments regarding finances is difficult. They often have trouble controlling their emotions, resulting in a short temper or frequent crying spells.

During the disease's early stages, the symptoms of Alzheimer's disease can usually be coped with—especially if family and friends are helpful. Forgetfulness can be overcome with gentle reminders and by keeping lists. Problems with thinking ability may require a trusted family member to help with finances. And communication problems aren't severe if people will be patient while talking and listening.

As the disease progresses, however, the changes will become more severe. Forgetfulness eventually reaches the point where lists aren't helpful—the affected person may not be able to remember to read the list. Dress and personal appearance become careless and routine household chores aren't performed. Some Alzheimer's victims may even forget to eat if not reminded. Living alone becomes so hazardous that an Alzheimer's sufferer will usually need to live with other members of the family.

Eventually the disease will affect communication and the ability to accomplish the most basic tasks such as turning on the television. A person in this stage of Alzheimer's disease will forget where they live and become totally lost if they wander from home. They may not recognize friends or even family members. Communication skills may deteriorate to the point that the person strings unrelated words into meaningless sentences. At this point, there is a need for constant supervision and nursing home care may become unavoidable.

Eventually, the failing nervous system affects all body functions. The person may be completely incapacitated—unable to walk or even eat.

What Causes Alzheimer's Disease?

Scientists have a clear understanding of the actual brain changes that are caused by Alzheimer's disease. In the simplest terms, Alzheimer's disease affects the brain tissue directly, causing neurons (nerve cells) to deteriorate and die. Because the brain cannot replace nerve cells, brain function is lost constantly throughout the course of the disease.

Although the exact cause of nerve cell destruction is not known, the way that the neurons die in Alzheimer's disease is unique. Abnormal structures called neurofibrillary tangles and senile plaques are found throughout the brains of people with Alzheimer's.

Plaques are the first change noted, sometimes occurring ten years or more before the first symptoms of Alzheimer's develop. The plaques are composed of a protein called amyloid beta. This protein is involved in the function of cell membranes and occurs normally in the brain in high concentrations. When plaques begin to develop, they consist of amyloid beta globules that collect in the spaces between the cells. As the globules begin collecting before any neurons begin to die, they are not simply protein left behind by dying cells.

Tangles consist of a different protein called tau. Normally, this protein forms into long fibers and rods inside the cell, providing structure and support for the cell. In Alzheimer's disease, the tau protein becomes twisted and tangled. It is possible that the tangled tau protein fibers damage the neurons. The neurofibrillary tangles may represent areas where abnormal tau protein has destroyed neurons.

As plaques and tangles accumulate in the brain, connections between nerve cells are reduced and neurons begin to die. It isn't certain, however, if the plaques and tangles themselves actually destroy the cells, or if they are a symptom of some other process that causes cell damage. In any case, plaques and tangles first form in the parts of the brain involved with short-term memory, which is not surprising considering that memory loss is one of the disease's first symptoms.

There are also changes in the neurotransmitters, the chemical messengers between the neurons. Levels of one of the most common neurotransmitters, acetylcholine, drop by up to 90 percent in the brains of Alzheimer's suffers. In all likelihood, the drop in neurotransmitter levels is caused by cell damage and destruction. It is therefore considered a symptom of the disease rather than a cause.

What events cause the brain to undergo these changes is not clearly understood. There is probably no single cause of Alzheimer's disease. However, research over the last few decades has found a variety of risk factors, that is, things that make a person more likely to develop Alzheimer's. Age is the greatest risk factor. Fewer than 2 percent of people under age sixty-five have the disease, while half of all people over age eighty-five have it. Women are more likely than men to develop Alzheimer's during their lifetime, although part of the increased risk women experience is because they live longer. The risk of developing Alzheimer's disease is about the same for all races and appears to be roughly the same in all parts of the world.

There are probably no environmental factors that contribute to developing Alzheimer's disease. At one point, researchers discovered that some Alzheimer's victims had small deposits of aluminum in their brain. Every known environmental source of aluminum, from antacids and antiperspirants to cookware, was then studied as a possible cause of the disease. None of the other studies have demonstrated any link between environmental aluminum and Alzheimer's disease. At this point, there does not seem to be any other environmental factor that increases the risk of developing Alzheimer's.

There is a genetic risk for developing Alzheimer's disease. Early onset Alzheimer's disease (prior to age sixty) is almost certainly a hereditary condition. There is also some genetic risk for developing the more common type of Alzheimer's disease, although the risk is not nearly as strong as for early onset Alzheimer's. A person with a family history of Alzheimer's disease is slightly more likely to develop it than a person with no family history. Even in families where several members have developed Alzheimer's, however, the majority of family members will not develop the disease.

Genetic research done as part of the Human Genome Project has begun to locate some of the exact genes that place people at risk of developing Alzheimer's disease. A single gene, known as ApoE, exists in many different forms in different people (similar to the single gene that can code for any of several different blood types). In the early 1990s, scientists discovered that people who have the E4 form of the ApoE gene are more likely to develop Alzheimer's disease after age sixty-five than people with other forms of the gene. Even so, most people who have the ApoE-4 gene do not develop Alzheimer's disease. In other words, having the ApoE-4 gene type puts a person at higher risk for developing Alzheimer's disease, but is not enough by itself to cause the disease. Clearly, there must be other factors besides this gene that contribute to the development of Alzheimer's.

In March of 1998 another new genetic association with Alzheimer's disease was reported. This gene, which is known as BH, also has several different forms. People with one form of BH are also more likely to develop Alzheimer's than people with other forms. Because the BH gene contains the genetic code for an enzyme involved in creating amyloid, a substance commonly found in the brain plaques of Alzheimer's patients, it may provide new clues about how the disease emanates.

Diagnosing Alzheimer's Disease

Unfortunately, the only way to be absolutely certain a person has Alzheimer's disease is to examine their brain at autopsy. Because this is not an option in living patients, doctors must diagnose the disease by exclusion, that is, by ruling out all other causes of a person's symptoms. The first step in diagnosing Alzheimer's is to insure that a person with some of the early symptoms really has dementia. This can often be accomplished simply by taking a history and administering a few bedside tests that evaluate brain function. In early cases, however, it may be necessary to administer some neuropsychological or mental status tests to evaluate exactly how well a person is thinking and remembering.

Doctors will also conduct tests to rule out other causes of dementia (Table 16.1). This almost always involves either an MRI or CT scan (see chapter 4) or both. An EEG (electroencephalogram, sometimes referred to as a brain wave test) may also be ordered. A general medical evaluation should be done to make certain the person does not have a systemic (involving the whole body) disease that could cause dementia such as thyroid problems or liver failure. A psychological evaluation may also be needed to be absolutely certain that depression isn't the cause of the problems. Depression in older people often becomes severe enough to cause mental disturbances similar to dementia.

When it has been proven that a person suffers dementia, and all of the other causes have been ruled out, doctors can accurately diagnose Alzheimer's disease 90 percent of the time. In the remaining cases it may be necessary to watch for slow and gradual changes in mental status and function before doctors are absolutely certain the person does, or does not, have Alzheimer's disease.

Unfortunately, it sometimes happens that an elderly person whose mental function is not what it once was is told they have Alzheimer's disease without a thorough evaluation. This can obviously have devastating emotional effects on the patient and their family. Before actually making the diagnosis of Alzheimer's disease, the doctor should be certain that all of the following are present:

1. Clearly established dementia, either absolutely obvious to others or confirmed by neuropsychological tests.
2. Progressive worsening of memory and thought processes over time.
3. No disturbance of consciousness.
4. Symptoms begin between the ages of forty and ninety.
5. No systemic disease or other brain disease that could explain the symptoms found.

Other factors that will help to further confirm the diagnosis of Alzheimer's disease include:

1. A family history of Alzheimer's disease.
2. Deterioration of specific functions (such as speech) over time.
3. Associated symptoms of depression, insomnia, delusions, hallucinations, emotional outbursts, and weight loss are present. (These symptoms usually do not occur until the late stages of Alzheimer's disease, however.)

TESTS FOR ALZHEIMER'S DISEASE

Obviously, it is difficult to be absolutely certain that a person has Alzheimer's disease until the symptoms are fairly advanced. Researchers are attempting to develop tests that will allow doctors to diagnose the disease early in its course. This would not only give patients and families early warning that the progressive disease is present, but could allow preventive and therapeutic treatments currently being developed to be started earlier.

One test that is often useful in making the diagnosis of Alzheimer's disease is Magnetic Resonance Imaging, or MRI (see chapter 4). The test is often used to be certain that other causes of dementia, such as multiple strokes or a brain tumor, are not present. The MRI can also reveal atrophy (shrinkage) of the brain tissue, which is present in patients with Alzheimer's disease and those with other neurodegenerative diseases. Newer high-resolution MRI equipment can also show if the atrophy is worse in the specific areas of the brain that are most severely affected by Alzheimer's disease, thus providing further evidence that the disease is present.

While they are still considered experimental tests, positron emission tomography (PET), single photon emission computed tomography (SPECT), and magnetic resonance spectroscopy imaging (MRSI) can all show doctors how the brain is working at a chemical level (see chapter 4). Alzheimer's disease causes some characteristic chemical changes that might be detected by these tests during the disease's very early stages. If research determines that this can be done accurately, SPECT and MRI scans could be employed with both greater frequency and effectiveness to diagnose Alzheimer's disease within the next several years. One study reports that PET scans can detect changes in people who will develop Alzheimer's disease years before they have any symptoms (remember, this is just one study that hasn't yet been confirmed). Because of the high cost and complexity of PET scans, however, there is little chance that they will become widely available in the near future.

Another type of test that may help to diagnose Alzheimer's disease with certainty is the detection of biological markers (certain body chemicals such as proteins) that are found only in people with the disease. Tests that measure the spinal fluid levels of amyloid beta protein (the protein in plaques), tau protein (the protein in tangles), and a third protein associated with Alzheimer's disease have recently been developed. Some of these tests are already available, but currently there is a great degree of controversy about their accuracy. At this time, most doctors believe these tests can help confirm the diagnosis of Alzheimer's disease when it is already suspected, but they are not yet foolproof enough to substitute for a complete evaluation.

Testing spinal fluid for tau protein is probably the most widely accepted biological marker test. Most (but not all) people with Alzheimer's disease have elevated levels of tau protein—even very early in the disease when symptoms are minimal. Tau levels remain high as the disease progresses, and are high no matter what age the patient was when they first developed symptoms. However, persons with certain other neurodegenerative diseases, and even people with dementia caused by multiple strokes, often have elevated tau protein levels. A similar test is available for beta amyloid peptide, but it is considered to be less accurate than the tau protein test.

A similar test of spinal fluid checks the level of a different protein called AD7C-NTP (if you want to make your doctors squirm ask them what AD7C-NTP stands for!). Although this test is still in the development stage, early results suggest it *may* be more accurate for detecting Alzheimer's disease than the tau protein test. (The AD7C-NTP test may be released by the time this book is available.)

A simple blood test is also available that detects if a person has the ApoE-4 gene, which is associated with a high risk of developing Alzheimer's (see page 283). Simply having this gene does not mean that a person has Alzheimer's, but the test may provide a bit more information that will help the doctor decide if a patient's dementia is caused by Alzheimer's. Most physicians agree that people should not take the test to see if they will develop Alzheimer's disease later in life. Most people who have the gene will not develop Alzheimer's disease, but a positive test might cause years of worry.

Unfortunately, the accuracy of ApoE-4 blood tests has recently been questioned. In 1997, a panel of experts at the National Institutes of Health stated that a blood tests for ApoE-4, which was developed by a single company, was more accurate than another, similar test. In 1998, it was found that this company had provided funding to organize the panel and that five members of the panel had financial ties to the company. While the panel's statement may be accurate, other competing companies, and some physicians, claim that the panel's conclusions were biased.

Treatment of Alzheimer's Disease

There is no cure for Alzheimer's disease. At this point there are not even treatments that are certain to slow progression of the disease. However, there is much reason for hope. Research in Alzheimer's treatments has literally exploded during the last five years.

New drugs have recently become available that can temporarily improve mental function in some people with mild Alzheimer's disease. Other research indicates that some treatments may delay onset of the disease in people at high risk. And research is continuing at a breakneck pace. At this time, early 1999, there are at least twenty-three different drugs for Alzheimer's disease that are in preliminary or clinical trials. Early results hint that many of them may be more effective than any of the medications currently available.

CAN YOU REDUCE THE RISK OF DEVELOPING ALZHEIMER'S DISEASE?

We know that the degeneration in the brains of Alzheimer's victims begins years before they exhibit any symptoms of the disease. Recent research has shown that several treatments may be effective in slowing this degeneration, especially if treatments are started before the onset of symptoms.

It needs to be stated, however, that some of these risk-reducing treatments are already being "hyped" far beyond their (probable) value. Because several of these treatments involve over-the-counter or herbal preparations, please be aware that a lot of people with no medical or neurological qualifications are already marketing these items as "Alzheimer's cures," particularly over the Internet. Some are probably sincere, and some are probably making a lot of money, but no evidence points to any of these treatments as "cures." There is only some early scientific data that suggests they slow progression of the disease.

Antioxidants

Antioxidants are substances that can bind free radicals, which are simply oxygen atoms that are missing an electron. Free radicals are very reactive chemicals, and will always combine with other molecules soon after they are formed. Because this chemical combination adds an oxygen atom to the molecule, it is called oxidation. (The oxidation of iron, for example, is commonly called rust.) Oxidation damages cells by destroying important molecules, including DNA, that the cell requires to function. Oxidation damage contributes to the development of certain cancers, is responsible for some of the effects of aging, and *may* be involved in the cellular damage present in Alzheimer's disease.

Free radicals are formed in the bodies of all animal life, either as a byproduct of normal metabolism, or because they are released by certain cells to perform specific functions. For example, some white blood cells release free radicals in areas of infection to kill bacteria. Normally the body contains certain chemicals, known as antioxidants, that trap most of the free radicals before they do much damage. Several vitamins, particularly vitamin E (also known as alpha-tocopherol), are very effective free radical trappers. (This is not vitamin E's only function; it also is needed to produce red blood cells and for the immune system to function properly.)

Evidence exists that free radicals play a role in Alzheimer's disease. The destruction of neurons involves some inflammation (chemical swelling) of brain tissue, and inflammation produces free radicals. Beta amyloid, the chemical that forms the senile plaques found in Alzheimer's patient's brains, reacts with the cells lining the brain's blood vessels. This reaction also produces a large amount of free radicals. Neurons are highly susceptible to free radical damage because brain tissue does not contain many antioxidant compounds.

Theoretically, antioxidants might help preserve neurons in Alzheimer's disease by absorbing free radicals before they can damage cells. Recent research does suggest that high doses of antioxidant compounds, particularly vitamin E and the medication selegiline (Eldepryl®), may slow progression of Alzheimer's disease.

One very thorough study, published in the *New England Journal of Medicine* in 1997, showed that Alzheimer's patients taking either selegiline or vitamin E were able to care for themselves slightly longer and progressed to severe dementia a bit more slowly than patients who did not take antioxidants. Interestingly, the drugs appeared to work better when one was taken alone rather than when both were taken in combination. Overall, the antioxidants only delayed the disease's progression by about seven months compared to its natural course, however.

A separate study performed by European researchers determined that selegiline improved memory during the early stages of Alzheimer's disease. Selegiline also enhanced the benefits of tacrine (Cognex®), one of two drugs currently approved for treating thought problems in persons with Alzheimer's disease.

Anti-inflammatory Drugs

As mentioned above, some evidence suggests that part of the damage occurring during Alzheimer's disease is caused by inflammation around the brain's cells. A few studies of families with a high frequency of Alzheimer's disease suggested that family members who took arthritis medication regularly were less likely to develop the disease than their siblings who didn't have arthritis. The drugs that seemed most effective were the nonsteroidal anti-inflammatory drugs (NSAIDs). These are inflammation-reducing drugs that don't contain cortisone or other steroids. Common NSAIDs include medications such as ibuprofen (Advil®, Motrin, Nuprin®), naproxen (Aleve®, Naprosyn®), and many others.

A long-term study (patients were followed for fifteen years!) released by the National Institute on Aging in 1997 showed that people who regularly took NSAIDs had a 30 to 50 percent lower risk of developing Alzheimer's disease than people who did not use these medications. It wasn't necessary to take the drugs for the entire fifteen years to obtain the beneficial effect. Those who only took the drugs for as little as two of the fifteen years showed a reduced risk. Using the drugs for a longer time period did result in a further reduction in Alzheimer's risk, however.

This long-term study eliminated several possible flaws that had made the earlier studies less convincing. It also gave researchers the chance to compare different types of anti-inflammatory medications to each other. While all the NSAIDs studied reduced the risk of Alzheimer's, acetaminophen (Tylenol) and aspirin had no benefit. This isn't surprising for Tylenol, since this drug has no anti-inflammatory activity, but it is surprising for aspirin, which is a potent anti-inflammatory drug.

Not only has this research pointed to a possible protective measure against Alzheimer's, it has also strengthened the theory that inflammation may be an important link in the Alzheimer's disease process. NSAID medications do cause some side effects, particularly stomach irritation and interference with kidney function to a slight degree, but they are generally very safe medications and are available over-the-counter.

Estrogen

It has been known for many years that women are slightly more likely to develop Alzheimer's disease than men. Researchers began to explore the effect of estrogen on Alzheimer's disease in the 1980s. Since then it has been reported that women who take estrogen replacement therapy regularly after menopause are 30 to 40 percent less likely to develop Alzheimer's disease than women who do not. Some doctors are recommending estrogen replacement in women with strong family histories of Alzheimer's disease.

A few studies seem to indicate that estrogen has a small beneficial effect on women who already have Alzheimer's disease. However, the studies that showed improvement involved only small groups of patients for a short time. Larger, more complete studies should be released within the next several years.

DRUGS USED TO TREAT ALZHEIMER'S DISEASE

In the last decade, researchers have discovered drugs that appear to improve memory and thinking ability in persons with Alzheimer's disease. A few animal studies even hint that we may soon find medications that can reverse some of the changes of the disease, or at least halt its progression. These implications are so exciting that the medications often receive a lot of publicity, even though the drugs themselves are in the earliest testing stages and won't be available for many years.

There are already some medications available that can help reduce the symptoms of Alzheimer's disease. A few new drugs may even improve memory and thinking ability, at least for a while. None of the drugs offers a cure for Alzheimer's, but they can improve the patient's condition, especially during the early and middle stages of the disease.

Before discussing medication that will help an Alzheimer's disease patient, however, it must be mentioned that some commonly used medications worsen the symptoms of the disease. For example, many prescription medications and over-the-counter drugs cause a little sedation. Most of us know what it feels like to be a bit "fuzzy headed" from a cold pill or other medication. When a person with Alzheimer's disease takes medication, this effect is magnified greatly. Even medications that they have taken for years without trouble can dramatically worsen their thought processes or memory.

In particular alcohol, some antidepressants, certain heart medications, cold and sinus medications, some blood pressure medicine, and especially tranquilizers can worsen the symptoms of Alzheimer's disease. The effects become magnified when several different medications are taken at the same time, a situation common in older people. Whenever an Alzheimer's patient is taking several medications, a doc-

Table 16.2 Some Medications Currently in Clinical Trials for Alzheimer's Disease

Medication	Claims	Contraindications	Side Effects
ENA-713 (Novartis Pharmaceuticals, applied for FDA approval)	The drug results in improvement of symptoms without the bad effects of Tacrine.	Uncertain at this time.	Nausea and vomiting occurred in 40 percent of patients taking the drug. Dizziness, fatigue, muscle aches, and urinary incontinence were also reported frequently with sweating and vision changes being reported less frequently.
Metrifonate (Bayer Pharmaceuticals, applied for FDA approval—the application is on hold pending review of a few severe respiratory problems)	Improves thinking and behavioral symptoms in mild Alzheimer's disease. One small study suggests that the compound may slow the deterioration rate in Alzheimer's disease. A study published in 1996 showed significant improvements in neuropsychological tests but no long-term or large studies have been performed.	Some heart conditions, glaucoma.	Occasional diarrhea, nausea, and leg cramps. The drug causes a slight decrease in heart rate.

Table 16.2 Some Medications Currently in Clinical Trials for Alzheimer's Disease (*continued*)

Medication	Claims	Contraindications	Side Effects
Idebenone (Avan®; currently in Phase II clinical trials)	Treatment for many dementias including Alzheimer's disease. The medication may improve thought processes and behavioral symptoms in mild to moderate dementia. Theoretically, it improves brain metabolism, provides protection for brain cells against certain types of destruction, and increases secretion of nerve growth factor, which helps stimulate new connections between neurons. Two large studies have shown positive effects.	Unknown.	Occasional nausea, headaches, dizziness, and bronchitis. The drug also may cause mild liver damage.
Propentyofylline (Hoechst Marion Roussel; currently in Phase III clinical Trials)	General improvement in mild to moderate dementia caused by Alzheimer's disease. A large, multicenter study showed the drug improves thinking and daily living skills in both Alzheimer's disease and vascular dementia.	Unknown.	Occasional nausea, dizziness, abdominal cramps, and headache.

Medication	Claims	Contraindications	Side Effects
Galanthamine (Reminyl™; Janssen Pharmaceutica; currently in Phase III clinical trials)	Improves thinking ability in mild to moderate Alzheimer's disease. One very early study showed the drug slowed deterioration in mental status for at least a year.	Unknown.	Occasional nausea and vomiting, particularly in the first few days.
Eptastigmine, MF-201 (Mediolanum Pharmaceuticals; currently in Phase III clinical trials)	Improves thought process in patients with Alzheimer's disease. A few studies show improvement for up to twenty-five weeks, but no large, long-term studies have been done.	Unknown.	Occasional agitation, insomnia, nausea, and dizziness.

Table 16.2 Some Medications Currently in Clinical Trials for Alzheimer's Disease (*continued*)

Medication	Claims	Contraindications	Side Effects
Xanomeline, LY 246708 (Eli Lilly; skin patch currently in Phase II clinical trials)	Improves thinking, behavioral emotional symptoms in patients with mild to moderate Alzheimer's disease. The drug originally developed in oral form that had to be discontinued because it caused digestive tract problems. It is now being tested in a skin patch form. A large, long-term study showed benefits in thinking with less agitation, hallucinations, and mood swings.	Unknown.	Causes slight anxiety in some people.
NeoTrofin, AIT-082 (NeoTherapeuticx Inc.; currently in Phase II clinical trials)	General improvement in mild to moderate Alzheimer's disease. It mimics the effects of nerve growth factor and other neurohormones. Theoretically, this might actually help patients with Alzheimer's disease, but this idea remains quite speculative at this time.	Probably contraindicated for patients with history of ulcer or heart disease.	Sweating , nausea, heartburn, and chills occur fairly frequently. Chest pain and fainting occur occasionally.

tor should carefully review them. It is often possible to reduce or change the patient's medication regimen to help improve their mental state.

Medications for Behavioral and Emotional Symptoms

Many people with Alzheimer's disease experience changes in their emotional state. A few begin behaving in dangerous or unacceptable ways, especially during the middle and latter stages of the disease. These changes not only cause problems for the affected person, they also cause stress and anxiety for those attempting to care for them. Medications can help control emotional and behavioral problems, and in some cases can make the difference between being able to care for the Alzheimer's sufferer at home and having to place them in a nursing home.

Risperidone (Risperdal®) is the medication most frequently used to treat behavioral problems, delusions, hallucinations and severe anxiety. Since these problems occur eventually in almost 40 percent of persons with Alzheimer's disease, this medication is commonly used. Risperidone reduces the severity and frequency of delusions and is very effective for treating agitation and anxiety. Reducing delusions and agitation often helps make behavior problems more manageable. Risperidone does not improve thinking, memory loss, or any other symptoms of Alzheimer's disease, however.

The major side effect of Risperidone is reduced blood pressure, especially when a person first stands up from a sitting position. This side effect occurs in almost one-third of people taking the drug and sometimes can result in fainting. The drug also causes mild sedation in most people but may prove heavily sedating in a few cases. Both sedation and blood pressure changes tend to clear up over time, however.

Severe agitation and behavioral problems that might result in harm to the patient or to others may require other antipsychotic medications (the "major" tranquilizers). Before prescribing potent antipsychotic medications for a behavioral problem, however, a doctor should evaluate the patient carefully for other causes. Sudden changes in behavior or agitation may occur when an Alzheimer's patient suffers pain, infection, dehydration, or even impaired vision or hearing. It isn't unusual for a patient in the latter stages of Alzheimer's to become severely agitated when they lose their glasses or if their hearing aid battery runs down. Like Risperidone, all the major tranquilizers can cause sedation or blood pressure reduction.

Less severe emotional problems that occur during Alzheimer's disease include depression, anxiety, and sleeplessness. The newer antidepressant medications can help relieve depression without worsening memory or thought processes. Certain antidepressants can also improve sleeping patterns and reduce agitation. Mild tranquilizers are sometimes required to treat anxiety and agitation, but these medications should be used sparingly since they will often worsen metal function. Medications that are used to improve thought processes in Alzheimer's disease patients may also help to relieve anxiety.

Medications for Cognitive (Thinking and Memory) Symptoms

One of the most exciting areas of medical research during the last ten years has been the development of medications that can actually improve memory, thinking, and reasoning in Alzheimer's disease patients. It has been known for many years that levels of the neurotransmitter acetylcholine are markedly reduced by Alzheimer's disease. Logically, doctors assumed that medications that either increased acetylcholine levels or mimicked acetylcholine's actions might help to treat Alzheimer's disease patients.

An enzyme called acetylcholine esterase, located at the synapse (the area of connection between two nerve cells), destroys acetylcholine immediately after it is released from a nerve ending. In order to negate this, researchers have developed drugs to prevent this enzyme from working, thereby increasing acetylcholine levels. Two such drugs have been released for the treatment of Alzheimer's disease: Donepezil (Aricept™) and Tacrine (Cognex). Many similar drugs are currently under development. While none of these drugs can cure

Alzheimer's disease, in some cases they can lessen its effects. Both drugs—currently on the market—are most effective during the early and middle stages of the disease.

Donepezil (Aricept)   Donepezil was approved for treatment of Alzheimer's disease in 1996. As mentioned, Donepezil works by inhibiting the enzyme acetylcholine esterase, which acts to break down acetylcholine after it has been released by a nerve cell. Acetylcholine esterase exists throughout the body, but Donepezil works only on the specific variety of the enzyme that is located in the brain. Because the medication does not affect acetylcholine esterase in the rest of the body, its side effects should be limited. Donepezil also has the advantage of requiring only a single dose each day, an important factor for people who may have difficulty remembering when they should take their medicine.

Alzheimer's patients often show improvement in their thought processes and behavior when taking Donepezil. In the largest study to date, patients taking the drug had significant improvement in thinking, short-term memory, and daily functioning for twenty-four weeks. It's still not certain how long the drugs will continue to prove beneficial, however, or even what percentage of patients will truly benefit from taking it.

Donepezil's side effects include nausea, diarrhea, loss of appetite, fatigue, and difficulty sleeping. None of them occur frequently, however. When they do occur, the side effects are usually mild and disappear within one to three weeks if the patient continues to take the medication.

Tacrine (Cognex™)   Tacrine was the first drug approved for Alzheimer's disease and has been available since 1993. Tacrine is an acetylcholine esterase inhibitor as is Donepezil. The difference is that Tacrine inhibits the enzyme both in the brain and throughout the body. Several different studies have shown that Tacrine improves mental function in 20 to 40 percent of people with Alzheimer's disease. It may even prove somewhat beneficial in moderately to severely advanced cases.

Because it inhibits the enzyme throughout the body, Tacrine causes more frequent and more severe side effects than Donepezil. Nausea, vomiting, diarrhea, abdominal pain, and skin rash have all been reported. The most common side effect, however, is an elevation of liver enzymes. Severe liver damage has been reported in a few cases. For this reason, people taking Tacrine must have blood tests to check liver function regularly.

The drug also must be taken four times a day, which can be a problem for some patients. Because the drug itself is fairly expensive and regular blood tests will be required during use, the cost of treatment using Tacrine may be prohibitive for some people. For those who benefit from Tacrine, though, its cost and side effects may be a minor issue compared to improved mental function.

Other Medications   Several promising new acetylcholine esterase inhibiting drugs are currently undergoing clinical trials and may be available within the next few years. Metrifonate, a new acetylcholine esterase inhibitor from Bayer Corporation, is probably the closest to receiving FDA approval, but is under review because of possible side effects. Like Donepezil, Metrifonate is taken just once a day and appears to have relatively few side effects. Other acetylcholine esterase inhibitors undergoing clinical tests include ENA-713 (Sandoz), Physostigmine SR (Forest), NXX-066 (Astra Arcus), and Galanthamine (Janssen).

A different class of medications actually increases production of acetylcholine rather than stopping its breakdown. Medications from this class currently in clinical trials include Xanomeline (Eli Lilly), Milameline (Parke-Davis), SB-202026 (SmithKline Beecham), AF-102B (Snow Brand Products), and ABT-418 (Abbott). It remains unclear whether these medications will be more or less effective than the acetylcholine esterase inhibitors. They may also prove useful in combination with those drugs. It is expected to be several years before the first acetylcholine-producing medications are available.

Another class of medications, called ampakines, may also improve memory in Alzheimer's patients through an entirely different mechanism. These medications do not work on acetylcholine at all, rather, they increase levels of a different neurotransmitter in the brain called AMPA-glutamate. Ampalex™, the first medication from the ampakine class, was tested in Germany and Sweden on fifty-four people with normal brain function. Compared to those not taking the drug, those test subjects using Ampalex scored twice as high on short-term memory tests. While the drug appears to improve memory and reasoning, it is unclear if it will benefit persons with Alzheimer's disease.

There are rapid advancements being made in other areas of Alzheimer's treatment. Within five years there may be a dozen different medications used to treat Alzheimer symptoms, compared to the two available currently. Table 16.2 contains more information about drugs currently undergoing clinical trials. If you are thinking of entering a clinical trial to gain access to one of these drugs, please read the section on clinical trials in chapter 13 first. If you are still interested, appendix D lists several organizations you can contact for more information.

OTHER MEASURES THAT MAY HELP ALZHEIMER'S PATIENTS

Ginkgo

Ginkgo, or *Ginkgo biloba*, refers to an extract from the leaves of the ginkgo tree, the oldest surviving species of tree on Earth. For years, herbalists have claimed that ginkgo can treat many conditions associated with aging, including memory loss. Recently, some medical studies have suggested it may help persons with Alzheimer's disease.

Medically, it has been proven that the active ingredient in ginkgo extract interferes with the action of a substance in the body called platelet activation factor (PAF). Platelet activation factor is involved in a number of different processes throughout the body. In Europe, where physicians are more likely to prescribe and study herbal remedies, several studies seem to indicate that the extract can have significant effects on the brain.

At least one study suggests that ginkgo extract helps restore blood flow through the brain in people with cerebral vascular disease. Patients participating in this study also reported that they believed their memory had improved. A British study suggested that even healthy young people had improved memory when taking ginkgo (although most physicians aren't very impressed with this study). A well-documented German study, however, determined that Alzheimer's and other dementia patients taking ginkgo had improved their thinking and reasoning ability as measured by standardized tests. The German food and drug administration has endorsed ginkgo for treatment of dementia.

More recently, American researchers have published studies that bolster the European research. A year-long study published in the *Journal of the American Medical Association* compared treatment with ginkgo to a placebo in patients with early dementia. The study concluded that patients taking ginkgo had improved mental function for periods of six months to one year.

It should be noted that even in the most optimistic study the effect of ginkgo was small. It is important to remember that herbal medicines are still medicines: they have side effects. Ginkgo can interfere with blood clotting, may cause allergic reactions, and some people report headaches or nausea when taking it.

Acetyl-L-Carnitine

Acetyl-l-carnitine, usually simply referred to as carnitine, is a nutritional supplement. Specifically, it is a combination of two amino acids (the building blocks of protein): lysine and methionine. A few studies have suggested that taking carnitine can slow the progression of Alzheimer's disease.

In the early 1990s, two studies gave either carnitine or a placebo to patients with Alzheimer's. Both studies found that patients continued to deteriorate, but the ones taking carnitine did not deteriorate as rapidly as those taking the placebo. A larger study completed in 1995 also found that Alzheimer's disease patients deteriorated at a slower rate if they were given carnitine. This latter study is considered more conclusive because the patients took a battery of neuropsychological tests that confirmed they had slower deterioration of mental function when they took carnitine.

As with ginkgo, the improvement was small and doctors are not absolutely certain that the treatment is effective. However, taken in reasonable doses (2,000 to 3,000 mg per day were used in the studies), carnitine causes few side effects except in patients with kidney disease. For this reason, most doctors do not object to patients taking it in addition to other medications.

MELATONIN

Melatonin is a hormone secreted naturally by the pineal gland in the brain. Its major known effect is in regulating the circadian, or sleep-wake cycle, and it is widely used as an over-the-counter treatment for insomnia. The sleep-wake cycle not only affects sleep, but also regulates several other functions including daily changes in body temperature and some hormone concentrations.

Melatonin levels decrease with age and fall even further in patients with Alzheimer's disease. It has been suggested that taking melatonin at bedtime might help to restore a more normal sleep-wake cycle in persons with Alzheimer's disease who often don't sleep well at night but are drowsy during the day. There are a few reports that conclude melatonin helps to restore a normal sleep-wake cycle in Alzheimer's sufferers, but there are others stating that it causes sleep patterns to be even worse, especially when taken in high doses.

While melatonin is sold over-the-counter in the U.S., in Europe it is regulated as a neurohormone and requires a prescription. Almost nothing is known about interactions between melatonin and other drugs and diseases, but because melatonin is a potent natural hormone, it may cause problems in some situations. While trial doses of melatonin are probably worthwhile in persons with severely disturbed sleep, it should be stopped at the first sign of worsening symptoms.

Other Treatments

Although drug treatments for Alzheimer's disease are becoming effective, the most important measures to help someone with Alzheimer's disease are simple, supportive tasks that seem rather obvious. Simple caretaking changes and support can result in a substantive improvement in the quality of life of an Alzheimer's patient compared to any medical therapy.

Perhaps the most important measure is education—not of the affected person but of family members. When family members know what to expect from the disease, they can better plan how to provide a safe environment for the Alzheimer's sufferer. Perhaps more importantly, the family can avoid a lot of frustration and anxiety, thus lowering their own stress level. There are local Alzheimer's support groups in almost every major city and in most medium-sized towns. For further reference see appendix D.

During the early and middle stages of the disease, most Alzheimer's patients remain either in their own home or in a family member's home. Overstimulation and understimulation should be avoided since it can increase anxiety and worsen symptoms. For example, loud music, lots of people in the house, and several conversations going on at once will overwhelm an Alzheimer's patient. On the other hand, dim lighting and being left alone may prove frightening to the Alzheimer's sufferer.

Change is also difficult for Alzheimer's patients. Moving them from one house to another, as some families must do to share caregiving, is certain to increase anxiety. When these moves are necessary, as many familiar objects as possible should be moved with the patient. Many families find that moving the patient's room furniture, so that they're surrounded by familiar things, dramatically reduces the stress of any move.

Every Alzheimer's sufferer will need help with planning and memory retention. A large calendar where each day's plans, chores, and activities are listed can be invaluable. Even regular routines such as bathing, dressing, and laundry may be forgotten if not written down. A bulletin board or marker board is usually better than a paper list because the latter can be easily misplaced or forgotten.

Planned, pleasurable activities can help prevent depression and improve quality of life. The patient may not be able to decide what they would like to do, but family members usually know what types of activities they enjoy. With a bit of planning and support, an Alzheimer's sufferer can usually enjoy life and avoid nursing home care for many years.

Other Causes of Dementia

There are literally dozens of other diseases and conditions that can cause dementia (see Table 16.1). While a few—particularly those caused by psychiatric or systemic diseases—can be cured, most can only be treated symptomatically, such as Alzheimer's disease.

VASCULAR DEMENTIA

Next to Alzheimer's disease, the most common cause of dementia is stroke. A single, large stroke rarely causes dementia. More commonly, several small strokes over time cause slow deterioration of brain function. As each stroke occurs, more brain tissue is lost until the affected person eventually develops dementia.

This type of dementia, known as multiple infarct dementia, usually happens in a stepwise fashion. Because the strokes are small, patients may ignore the minor neurologic problems that occur with each one. After a week or two, the symptoms improve until the next ministroke occurs. Often, the patient forgets about the minor numbness or weakness that passed, but eventually other people will notice deterioration in their mental function.

People with vascular dementia usually have some weakness or loss of sensation in parts of their body, something that doesn't occur in the other types of dementia. An MRI scan will show the old strokes and can diagnose the dementia. Because the brain tissue has been permanently destroyed by the strokes, however, the condition is irreversible. The good news is that treatment can often prevent further strokes from occurring.

PARKINSON'S DISEASE AND LEWY BODY DEMENTIA

Parkinson's disease is one of the most common neurodegenerative diseases (see chapter 17). About one-third of people with Parkinson's disease will develop dementia during the later phases of the disease. Interestingly, during the late stages of Alzheimer's some patients will develop some symptoms similar to those of Parkinson's disease.

In recent years, researchers have discovered a new type of dementia that is currently called Lewy body dementia. Lewy bodies are the abnormal areas of protein deposit and deterioration that occur in certain brain areas of Parkinson's disease patients. Autopsy studies have found that some people with dementia have Lewy bodies deposited throughout their brain—not just in the specific areas where they occur in Parkinson's disease.

In fact, some researchers now believe that Lewy body dementia is actually one of the most common causes of dementia. If this is true, then many people who actually have Lewy body dementia are misdiagnosed as having Alzheimer's disease. (Note: Lewy bodies can only be found during an autopsy examination.)

There are differences, however, between Lewy body dementia and Alzheimer's disease. Lewy body dementia usually has a more variable course than Alzheimer's disease, including episodes of severe confusion and periods when the person appears nearly normal. Hallucinations are also much more common in Lewy body dementia than Alzheimer's disease. At this point, however, treatment for the two conditions is the same.

CREUTZFELDT-JAKOB DISEASE AND "MAD COW" DISEASE

Creutzfeldt-Jakob disease is a rare and fatal brain disorder thought to be caused by a prion, a poorly understood type of protein that behaves much the same as a virus. The earliest symptoms of the disease are memory lapses, changes in behavior, and difficulty thinking. As the disease progresses, mental function deteriorates rapidly, sudden, uncontrollable jerking movements occur, and generalized weakness develops. Eventually blindness, coma, and death result. The disease can be transmitted from one person to another by blood transfusion or organ transplantation. There is evidence that "mad cow" disease is the same as, or very similar to, Creutzfeldt-Jakob disease. There is absolutely no treatment for Creutzfeldt-Jakob disease.

HUNTINGTON'S DISEASE

Huntington's disease (also known as Huntington's chorea or "Woody Guthrie's disease") is a neurodegenerative disease that usually begins in the mid-forties. The disease is a genetic disorder that causes brain cells in certain parts of the brain (known as the basal ganglia), to die.

Early in its course, patients notice abnormal, uncontrollable movements. As the disease progresses, intellect, memory, speech, and thought processes deteriorate. Eventually dementia develops.

There is no treatment for Huntington's disease, but a genetic test is available to detect if a person has inherited the gene from one of their parents. Anyone who carries the gene will invariably develop the disease and will pass it on to half of their children.

CHAPTER 17

Parkinsonism and Movement Disorders

Parkinsonism is actually a syndrome (a set of symptoms occurring together) that has several different causes. The three major symptoms of Parkinsonism are a tremor (shaking), muscular stiffness or rigidity, and slow movements. Additionally, many people with the condition also walk with short shuffling steps and have a stooped posture. They may speak in a soft, monotone voice, and often don't make normal gestures or change facial expressions while talking.

The tremor of Parkinsonism usually affects the hands and feet, but it can sometimes affect the entire body. It is referred to as a resting tremor because it is very obvious when the affected person is sitting still, but disappears when they make a purposeful movement. The stiffness is referred to as plastic rigidity because the person's muscles can be moved, yet always resist the movement to some degree. When doctors try to move the patient's arms and legs, the resistance feels like trying to bend a soft piece of plastic.

All Parkinsonism's symptoms are caused by damage to an area of the brain stem called the substantia nigra. The name means "black substance" in Latin, because this area of the brain has a deep black color when examined at autopsy, while the rest of the brain appears light tan or gray. The cells in the substantia nigra send branches to an area of the cerebral hemisphere called the corpus striatum, which in turn connects to several of the movement centers in the brain.

The cells in the substantia nigra manufacture the neurotransmitter dopamine, which they release to stimulate neurons in the corpus striatum. If the cells are damaged or don't produce and release dopamine properly for any reason, Parkinsonism results. It is not surprising, therefore, that Parkinsonism has several causes.

The chances of developing Parkinsonism increase with age. The disease is almost never observed in people less than forty years old, and only about 3 in every 1,000 between ages fifty-five to sixty-four have Parkinsonism. The incidence increases to 10 per 1,000 people between ages sixty-five and seventy-four, 30 per 1,000 people between the ages seventy-five to eighty-four, and 43 per 1,000 people age eighty-five and older. Overall, about 500,000 people in the U.S. suffer from Parkinsonism. The disease affects men and women equally.

Causes of Parkinsonism and Parkinson's Disease

Parkinson's disease and Parkinsonism are two terms that are often used interchangeably since both describe patients who have the symptoms described above: resting tremor, muscular rigidity, slow movements, and gait disturbance. Medically, Parkinsonism refers to any and all conditions that cause this set of symptoms. Parkinson's disease is one form (probably the most common form) of Parkinsonism, but it can also be caused by many other conditions (Table 17.1).

In Parkinson's disease, patients have loss of pigmented neurons in the substantia nigra, and if the brain tissue is examined under a microscope the cells contain reddish lumps called Lewy bodies. In other forms of Parkinsonism patients have the same signs and symptoms, and may (or may not) have loss of the pigmented neurons in the substantia nigra. The other forms of Parkinsonism usually do not develop Lewy bodies. However, because Lewy bodies can only be found at autopsy, the diagnosis of Parkinson's disease is made by clinical symptoms.

Parkinson's disease is the most common form of Parkinsonism. Its cause is not known. Environmental factors don't appear to play any role in the development of Parkinson's disease. The problem occurs with the same frequency in almost every country in the world and was just as common in the late 1800s as it is today.

There is probably a genetic risk for developing Parkinson's disease since almost half the people with it have an ancestor or blood relative who also has it. Recent research at the National Institutes of Health has found at least one gene, coding for a protein called alpha synuclein, that causes one form of hereditary Parkinson's disease. Although the alpha synuclein gene causes only this one form of Parkinsonism, it is expected that other Parkinsonism genes will be discovered in the near future. While genetics may place a person at risk of developing Parkinson's disease, even the close relatives of a person with the disease have less than a 10 percent chance of developing the disease themselves.

Many of the other forms of Parkinsonism have a known cause (see Table 17.1 on page 312). For example, several types of drugs can cause Parkinsonism. Most cases of drug-induced Parkinsonism are temporary; the symptoms go away once the drug is stopped. Some chemical toxins can cause permanent Parkinsonism, however. For example, MPTP (the abbreviation for a twelve-syllable chemical), a contaminant of some street drugs sold in 1982, caused permanent Parkinsonism in a few dozen people. Some people who survived poisoning with cyanide or other chemicals have also developed permanent Parkinsonism.

The condition has also been reported after a rare brain infection known as von Economo's encephalitis. Physical damage to the

Table 17.1   Conditions That Can Cause Parkinsonism

Viral encephalitis–von Economo's disease

Drugs (drug-induced Parkinsonism is usually reversible when the drug is
stopped)
    Neuroleptic medications (major tranquilizers, such as thorazine)
    Reserpine

Toxins
    MPTP
    Manganese
    Carbon monoxide
    Carbon disulfide
    Cyanide

Metabolic Conditions
    Hypothyroidism (low thyroid)
    Hypoparathyroidism

Degenerative Neurologic Diseases
    Bilateral striopallidodentate calcinosis (Fahr disease)
    Diffuse Lewy body disease
    Wilson's disease
    Shy-Drager syndrome
    Olivopontocerebellar atrophy
    Progressive supranuclear palsy
    Striatonigral degeneration

substantia nigra can also cause Parkinsonism. In very rare cases, the
physical damage is caused by a stroke or tumor, but in far more cases
the damage is caused by repeated minor head injuries. Boxers who become "punch drunk," for example, sometimes are actually suffering
from a minor form of Parkinsonism. Certain rare diseases of the
brain, such as Shy-Drager syndrome and progressive supranuclear
palsy, can also cause Parkinsonism if they involve the substantia nigra.

In any case, the difference between Parkinsonism and Parkinson's
disease really doesn't have any effect on the patient. The symptoms

and treatment remain the same for all types of Parkinsonism. In the rest of this chapter, I will use the term *Parkinsonism* when describing all forms of the disease unless I'm specifically discussing Parkinson's disease.

Major Symptoms of Parkinsonism

The symptoms of Parkinson's disease appear slowly, often beginning several years before a person actually seeks medical treatment. Most other forms of Parkinsonism begin just as slowly, although cases that are caused by poisoning or injury will begin suddenly.

The early symptoms are usually nonspecific and mild. Family members may notice the affected person has a stooped posture or a bit of difficulty walking but often just assume it is a normal change caused by aging. The affected person may feel tired or just not well. In some cases, they may notice that they aren't thinking as clearly as usual, or are moving stiffly. Handwriting may also change, becoming small and scrawled. Because the early symptoms could be caused by a variety of other conditions, few doctors will even suspect Parkinsonism as a cause.

As the disease progresses, a tremor becomes noticeable, particularly when the person is tired or under stress. Handwriting changes may become severe; often it develops the unusual characteristic of getting smaller and smaller as the person continues to write a paragraph or two. The other characteristic symptoms, including muscle stiffness and slowness, usually become evident at this stage. Tremor and stiffness may only affect one limb, however.

At this stage, a doctor usually suspects Parkinsonism and may order several tests. None of them will show definitively that a person has Parkinsonism; their purpose is to insure that no other neurologic disease is causing the problem. If tests rule out any other cause, doctors will state the person probably has Parkinsonism and begin treatment. Over time, the Parkinsonism's classic symptoms will become more apparent and the diagnosis will be made. The symptoms may remain mild for several years, however.

As symptoms progress, the affected person is said to have classic Parkinsonism. In this stage some degree of resting tremor is apparent. The severity of tremor may vary, being worse when the affected person is tired or stressed. It usually disappears during sleep and may only be obvious during times of stress or fatigue. The tremor will also get better and worse at random intervals, which may last anywhere from hours to weeks.

Stiffness and rigidity are often more noticeable to the doctor during examination than to the patient or family members during everyday, routine activities. Patients may be aware of muscle aching or cramps, and the tight muscles may cause a headache or pain in the shoulders and neck. The aches really don't get better with aspirin or Tylenol, but may be relieved by heat or massage.

The slowed movements caused by the disease are usually most noticeable to the patient. Automatic movements such as facial expressions, swinging the arms while walking, even eyeblinking and swallowing saliva, are all decreased by Parkinsonism. Voluntary movements may slow in several ways, although they seem less affected than automatic movements. In some cases, slowing becomes apparent as a delay between deciding to perform a movement and actually performing it. At other times, the movement begins normally but then slows and stops before it is completed. This is especially common with repeated movements such as walking. For example, someone with Parkinsonism may begin walking normally but their stride becomes shorter and slower after they've taken several steps.

Other symptoms occur in some cases. Soreness and muscle aches are common but usually not severe. Some patients experience frequent bouts of muscle cramps that are quite painful, while some find they can speak only in a soft, monotone voice. A few have difficulty swallowing. Constipation is also a problem for most people with

Parkinsonism, and a few have bladder or sexual difficulties. Excessive sweating also occurs in some cases, and burning, irritated eyes can also be a problem.

Changes in posture, especially bending forward while walking, are quite common in Parkinsonism. Most patients walk with short steps and don't lift their feet very high when they walk, resulting in a shuffling gait. In most cases this is noticeable, but the person can still walk without difficulty. During the late stages of the disease, however, some people experience severe trouble walking. Steps may be only a few inches at a time, they may have trouble balancing while walking, or occasionally may "freeze" every few steps.

Rare problems include difficulty reading because the muscles of the eyes don't function properly, low blood pressure, and oily skin. A few people also develop swelling in their legs and feet, although this is usually not severe. Many people with Parkinsonism also have bouts of depression, but this is severe in only a few cases.

While many patients exhibit all the classic symptoms of Parkinsonism, there seem to be two subgroups that are somewhat different. One group of patients suffers from slow movements and rigidity but has almost no tremor. These people tend to be older when they first develop Parkinsonism. As time passes they tend to have more trouble with posture and movement, and perhaps more intellectual problems, too. Another group of patients tends to have more tremor, but less rigidity and trouble with posture. Persons in this group tend to be younger when the disease develops but experience slower progression.

In most cases, the symptoms of Parkinsonism are well controlled by medications for years. Eventually, however, the symptoms become so severe that the medications no longer work well. In this late stage of Parkinsonism, the brain generally becomes more affected (Table 17.2, page 317). At this point, many patients have difficulty thinking properly, similar to the changes observed with Alzheimer's disease. This may progress to actual dementia (loss of contact with reality) and inability to care for themselves.

Secondary Symptoms of Parkinsonism

In addition to the major symptoms of Parkinsonism, many people will suffer one or more of the less common symptoms of the disease.

CONSTIPATION

Constipation is a problem for most Parkinsonism patients. Constipation is caused partially by chronic tightness of the pelvic muscles, and partially because the bowel does not seem to contract properly. Bulk fiber laxatives (Metamucil®, etc.) and high-fiber diets do not seem to help. Mild stimulant laxatives do help, but should probably be prescribed by your doctor so that he or she is aware of the problem. Taking too many stimulant laxatives will only worsen the problem over the long term.

SLEEP DISTURBANCE

Almost all patients with Parkinsonism report some difficulty sleeping. The most common problems are minor ones such as an inability to turn over or needing to use the bathroom during the night. About one-third of Parkinsonism patients have serious problems sleeping, however.

Some patients report they have a difficult time falling asleep due to the symptoms of the disease. Muscle aches and stiffness can make it difficult to find a comfortable sleeping position, or tremor may make it difficult to fall asleep (although the tremor disappears once sleep begins). Levodopa and other medications used to treat Parkinsonism are stimulants and may add to the difficulty of falling asleep. The medications can also cause nightmares or vivid dreams, resulting in patients waking up in the middle of the night.

Unfortunately, standard sleeping tablets often exacerbate muscle slowness. Benadryl® is often effective, however, and also helps tremor

Table 17.2   The Stages of Parkinsonism*

Stage One
   Signs and symptoms on one side only
   Symptoms are mild and inconvenient, but not disabling
   Usually presents with tremor of one limb
   Friends have noticed changes in posture, locomotion, and facial
      expression

Stage Two
   Symptoms on both sides
   Minimal disability but can perform everyday activities
   Posture and gait are affected

Stage Three
   Significant slowing of body movements
   Mild impairment of balance when walking or standing
   Some disability that is moderately severe

Stage Four
   Severe symptoms
   Can still walk but only to a limited extent
   Marked rigidity and slow movement
   No longer able to live alone
   Tremor may be less than at earlier stages

Stage Five
   Difficulty eating
   Cannot stand or walk
   Requires constant nursing care

This rating system is based on the Hoehn and Yahr Staging of Parkinson's Disease.

symptoms in some people. Changing the medication schedule to avoid stimulants during the evening can also help. Certain antidepressant medicines taken at bedtime often help patients to both fall asleep and remain asleep throughout the night.

Many patients with Parkinsonism (and their spouses) also complain that they are sleepy during the day and will fall asleep while watching television or sitting. Doctors are still not certain of the cause of daytime sleepiness. Not sleeping well at night certainly contributes to daytime sleepiness. Depression may also contribute, as can some of the medications required to treat the disease.

It does appear however, that Parkinsonism itself causes some degree of daytime sleepiness even after a good night's sleep. Treating daytime sleepiness has proven difficult. Stimulants, such as Ritalin or amphetamines help a few people, but often worsen anxiety and tremor. Some people report that the anti-Parkinson medication selegiline (see page 326) helps the problem without worsening other symptoms.

DEPRESSION

Almost half of all people suffering from Parkinsonism become clinically depressed. Common symptoms include worrying, withdrawal from social activities, insomnia, loss of interest in hobbies and other activities, loss of sex drive, and even thoughts of suicide. While some of the depression is an expected response to having a chronic disease, most doctors agree that Parkinsonism itself can cause depression as one of its symptoms.

Mild depression does not require any treatment except support from family and friends, but when depression becomes severe, it should be treated with medication. Medications for depression generally do not interfere with anti-Parkinson drugs and work just as well in Parkinsonism patients as in others.

DIZZINESS

Dizziness itself is not a symptom. However, many Parkinsonism patients feel unsteady when they walk and interpret this as being dizzy. Lightheadedness can also occur if medications lower blood pressure significantly, especially when standing up from a sitting position. In most cases, medication adjustments can be made to eliminate this problem.

DROOLING AND SWALLOWING PROBLEMS

Dysphagia, or difficulty swallowing, can occur if there is rigidity of the muscles of the throat and tongue. The same anti-Parkinson treatments that help muscles in other parts of the body will usually also help dysphagia. Swallowing problems can become severe in the late stages of the disease, however, causing pneumonia and difficulty when eating.

A few patients with Parkinsonism are embarrassed by a tendency to drool. This is because the muscles of the throat and tongue don't work properly, and the automatic swallowing reflex is impaired by the disease. No medications are very effective in controlling drooling, although there are a few that decrease saliva production.

DEMENTIA AND HALLUCINATIONS

Dementia (impaired thinking to the point that where there is loss of contact with reality) occurs in some people during the late stages of Parkinsonism. It is more common in those whose Parkinsonism is caused by another neurological disease (see Table 17.1 on page 312) such as olivopontocerebellar atrophy or progressive supranuclear palsy. It is also more common in patients older than age seventy.

When dementia does occur, it may take the form of grossly impaired thinking, extreme difficulty with memory, or even hallucinations. Dementia resulting from Parkinsonism is often associated with visual hallucinations. While these can be quite bizarre, and even frightening, they do not require any specific treatment. Some patients become quite agitated during hallucinations, however. In this case, tranquilizers will both reduce the frequency of hallucinations and reduce the agitation they cause. A few patients with dementia have "sundown syndrome" in which they become agitated and have hallucinations with the onset of evening.

The attending doctors should make a careful assessment to determine how severe the dementia is and insure it is not caused by a second disease other than Parkinsonism. Many Parkinsonism patients with early dementia are actually suffering from medication toxicity or other neurologic problems. Severe depression can also impair thinking and memory to the point where it appears similar to dementia. Dramatic improvement occurs when antidepressants are prescribed.

Most doctors will suggest reducing medications when dementia occurs—even if it should make the other symptoms of Parkinsonism worse. If the affected person is also agitated or violent to himself or others, tranquilizing medication will be required. Unfortunately, most Parkinsonism patients who develop dementia will require nursing home care. The drug clozapine (Clozaril®) may be effective in treating dementia caused by Parkinsonism. The drug can lower white blood cell counts in some patients, however, so a blood count must be checked every month when taking this medication.

Treatment of Parkinsonism

The treatment of Parkinsonism and Parkinson's disease is mostly symptomatic. That is, there are many medications that can reduce or relieve its symptoms, but there are no existing treatments that can reverse the damage or even halt progression of the disease. There are some experimental treatments (discussed below) that *may* at least slow the progression of the disease, but there remains a great deal of argument about whether they truly work.

PRINCIPLES OF MEDICATION THERAPY

Medical therapy of Parkinsonism is based on correcting the balance between two neurotransmitters (chemical messengers) in the brain: dopamine and acetylcholine. In most parts of the brain, these two neurotransmitters have opposite effects. In the normal brain a balance between dopamine and acetylcholine prevents the symptoms of Parkinsonism.

As mentioned earlier, people with Parkinsonism have low levels of dopamine in certain parts of their brain. Many of the medications used to treat the disease work by either increasing the levels of dopamine, or by imitating the action of dopamine. These medications are called dopaminergic (meaning dopamine-like) drugs.

Although patients with Parkinsonism have normal levels of acetylcholine, the proportion of acetylcholine to dopamine is higher than normal. A few drugs, known as anticholinergic drugs used to treat Parkinsonism, work by blocking acetylcholine. Blocking acetylcholine should restore the balance between acetylcholine and dopamine to a more normal level.

Treatment of Parkinsonism must be individualized for each patient and must be adjusted during the course of the disease. It is extremely important to realize that medical therapy has limitations and that the goal of treatment is to improve the symptoms, not eliminate them entirely. Often, the initial treatment improves symptoms dramatically, leaving only a little bit of tremor or stiffness.

Not surprisingly, most people want to take just a little more medicine to eliminate that last bit of tremor. The reality is that it takes more medicine to get rid of the last remaining bit of tremor than it did to stop the first 90 percent of it. Most of the anti-Parkinson medications have far more side effects at high doses, and it is likely that a person will develop significant medication side effects before they can rid themselves of the remaining Parkinsonism symptoms. It is also possible that taking higher doses of the medicine will shorten the amount of time the medication will remain effective. Given that the disease will slowly progress for years it can be important not to "run through" all the available medications during the first few years of treatment.

It's important, therefore, that patient, family, and physician all discuss and plan what the reasonable goals of medical therapy are at each stage of the disease. The general goal is to always obtain a reasonable improvement in symptoms while using the fewest drugs as infrequently as possible. During the early stages of Parkinsonism, it is often possible to relieve almost all the symptoms—except a bit of tremor or stiffness—with a single medication. Years later, a reasonable goal may be to remove 75 percent of the symptoms, leaving a person quite capable of caring for themselves but having some tremor and perhaps trouble walking normally. In the latest stages (often fifteen to twenty years after diagnosis), it may take several medications just to allow a person to perform everyday activities.

The best choice of medications varies for each individual with Parkinsonism. In most cases, at least one medication that increases levels of dopamine is used, although this may not be necessary in the very early stages of the disease. Additional medications may be used as certain symptoms become more severe, or if the original medications begin to lose effectiveness.

MEDICATIONS THAT INCREASE DOPAMINE

The therapy mainstay for Parkinsonism is the drug levodopa. Levodopa is a naturally occurring chemical (it's found in high concentration in fava beans) that neurons can easily convert to dopamine. (In case you're interested, taking dopamine by mouth does not help because it can't cross the blood–brain barrier.) Neurons can convert levodopa to dopamine much more easily than they can create dopamine "from scratch," so taking this medication increases the level of dopamine throughout the substantia nigra.

It takes some time for the levodopa to replenish stores of dopamine in the neurons, so the beneficial effects of the medication will build up over several days or even a week or two. After taking levodopa for a few days, most patients find that their movements speed up and their stiffness is reduced. Often voice and facial expressions return to normal. Patients usually feel more alert and seem to think more quickly. Tremor is not helped a great deal by levodopa, however.

Because levodopa is converted to dopamine throughout the body, only a small amount of the medication actually reaches the brain. For this reason, levodopa is often given in a combination pill that also contains the drug carbidopa (the combination pill is known as Sinemet®). The carbidopa prevents levodopa from being converted to dopamine by the body's cells. Since carbidopa doesn't cross the blood–brain barrier, only the brain can use levodopa effectively. In practice, a person only has to take about one-fifth as much levodopa when taken in combination with carbidopa. A similar drug, Madopar®, combines levodopa with a different inhibitor, with similar effects.

Levodopa can have a significant number of side effects, but they are usually manageable. The most common side effect is abnormal, involuntary movements that are known as dyskinesia. These movements may comprise simple fidgeting or occasional twitching, but in some cases turn severe with writhing movements, abnormal postures, and cramps present.

This side effect becomes increasingly common later in the disease when higher doses are required, but does occur in some people, especially women, even at low doses. It also becomes increasingly common when levodopa and a dopamine-like drug (see the following section) are taken together. There is no treatment that prevents this side effect, but sometimes it can be lessened by taking a time-release (long-acting) form of levodopa. Of course, the symptom will stop if levodopa is stopped, but most patients will tolerate the involuntary movement rather than suffer the return of their Parkinsonism symptoms.

Levodopa also has several effects on the brain other than improvement in Parkinsonism symptoms. It can also cause vomiting because it stimulates the brain's vomiting center; combining it with carbidopa usually prevents this side effect. It also causes nervousness or difficulty in sleeping for some people. This usually goes away after a few weeks of treatment. In a few cases, people become almost manic while taking levodopa, talking rapidly and constantly, and moving about while being unable to stay still. Small doses of tranquilizers will usually stop this side effect. Some people report vivid dreams or nightmares when beginning the medication. Levodopa can also interfere with the centers of the brain controlling blood pressure and heart functions. This can cause episodes of rapid heartbeat or may result in low blood pressure, especially when standing up from a sitting position.

People taking levodopa must also be careful about the other medications they take. The most severe interaction occurs between levodopa and a type of antidepressant medication called an MAO inhibitor. These antidepressants work by blocking an enzyme in the body called monamine oxidase (MAO), which breaks down dopamine, among other actions. Taking an MAO inhibitor together with levodopa can cause episodes of severely high blood pressure. A few other medications, notably vitamin B_6 and the antinausea drug Reglan®, can interfere with the beneficial effects of levodopa.

Despite its side effects, levodopa remains the most effective drug for treating Parkinsonism. Over time, however, it becomes less effective probably because fewer and fewer neurons are available to convert it to dopamine and then release the dopamine in the proper locations. In Parkinsonism's latter stages, levodopa may have to be taken every few hours. In other cases, it may be only minimally effective even when taken in high doses.

MEDICATIONS THAT MIMIC DOPAMINE

Since a lack of dopamine in certain areas of the brain causes Parkinsonism, it stands to reason that medications that act similarly to dopamine could relieve its symptoms. Over the years, dozens of medications known to have dopamine-like effects have been tried in patients with Parkinsonism, but the majority have been abandoned because they were either not effective or caused severe side effects. Two drugs of this type, bromocriptine (Pardolel®) and pergolide (Permax®) have been found effective against Parkinsonism, however.

Next to levodopa and carbidopa, these two drugs are the most effective medications for controlling Parkinsonism's symptoms. In general, they are about half as effective as levodopa and have fewer side effects. They may be used as the only treatment in early Parkinsonism, but the addition of levodopa will eventually be necessary. They may also be used late in the course of the disease to supplement the effects of levodopa. Of the two, pergolide works faster and has a longer duration of action than bromocriptine. But an individual may respond better to one medication than the other.

The side effects of pergolide and bromocriptine are almost identical. Many people experience nausea when beginning these drugs, but it will usually disappear if they can tolerate the medication for a few days. Lowered blood pressure, involuntary movements, vivid dreams, and nervousness may also occur. A very few people have experienced delusions and paranoia when taking these drugs. Bromocriptine can also activate peptic ulcer disease in people who have had an ulcer in the past. Both drugs can cause a discoloration of the skin or worsen angina (chest pain from coronary artery disease) in rare cases.

MEDICATIONS FOR TREMOR

For some patients with Parkinsonism, tremor is the major symptom and can become almost incapacitating. Since levodopa and the dopamine-like drugs do not reduce the tremor, other medications must be given specifically for tremor. Propranolol—a drug that blocks some of the effects of epinephrine (adrenaline)—is the most commonly used medication. It will generally reduce the amount of tremor by approximately 70 percent during Parkinsonism's early stages. Since this drug is available in a long-acting formula, it can often be given just once a day. People with bronchial asthma, congestive heart failure, and certain other conditions should not take propranolol, however. It can also cause depression.

People who cannot take propranolol are usually started on one of the anticholinergic drugs (see page 321) such as Artane® or Cogentin®. Some antihistamines, including Benadryl, are also effective in reducing tremor. None of these drugs are as effective as propranolol, however, usually resulting in only a 25 to 50 percent reduction in tremor.

Anticholinergic drugs have more side effects than propranolol. Most people experience dry mouth while taking these medications and many people have difficulty urinating. These drugs can also cause confusion or memory lapses in some people, especially those who already report difficulty in thinking as one of their symptoms.

If the tremor seems worse during periods of stress or anxiety, one of the tranquilizing medicines such as diazepam (Valium) or alprazolam (Xanax) may be effective. Tranquilizers often increase the slowness of movement in Parkinsonism patients, however, and are usually avoided for that reason.

Persons who have severe tremor that cannot be controlled by medications may have no choice but to consider surgery (see page 328–329). Only a few Parkinsonism patients ever develop tremor of this severity, however.

OTHER MEDICATIONS

Amantadine (Symmetrel®) is a medication sometimes used to protect against certain flu viruses. It was discovered by accident that the drug also imparts some generalized anti-Parkinson effects. Patients often note that their tremor is reduced, they feel better and more alert, and they move better. Doctors are continually debating exactly how the drug works in Parkinsonism, but all agree that it does work. It is sometimes used alone to treat early, mild symptoms since it is relatively inexpensive and has few side effects. It may also be used in addition to other drugs later in the course of disease.

Amantadine does impart side effects, including dry mouth, blurred vision, and constipation. In a few cases it causes a purple discoloration of the legs due to blood pooling in the small veins. Some people also find that amantadine loses its effectiveness after a few months. If they stop the drug for a few weeks and then restart it, however, its effectiveness will return.

Selegiline is one of the MAO inhibiting antidepressants. It works on only one subtype of MAO called MAO-B, however, which only metabolizes dopamine inside the brain. Persons taking levodopa can therefore safely take selegiline. In fact, selegiline enhances the effects of levodopa (both the good effects and the side effects) and prolongs its action.

Studies in the early 1980s showed that selegiline reduced the symptoms of Parkinsonism, even when taken without levodopa. It also prevented certain forms of drug-induced Parkinsonism in laboratory animals. This led researchers to speculate that selegiline might have a protective effect against Parkinsonism.

Human studies show that using the drug during early treatment may delay the time until levodopa will be needed, but amantadine and other medications do this also. At this time, whether selegiline actually slows the progression of Parkinsonism is still being debated, but most doctors do not believe that it does. Because selegiline is much more expensive than other anti-Parkinson medications, many doctors don't prescribe it very frequently. Others believe that even a small chance that it will delay the progression of the disease bodes in favor of taking selegiline.

CAST STUDY: Parkinsonism

William, a fifty-seven-year-old teacher, began to notice he felt much more tired than usual. He also began to feel stiff when he moved, a symptom he attributed to a bit of arthritis. He had two complete checkups but his doctor pronounced him in perfect health. During the next year, he noticed that when grading papers, his handwriting seemed small and difficult to read the longer he worked. He also developed a small tremor in his right hand.

He returned to his doctor who referred him to a neurosurgeon to see if there was a problem with the nerves in his hand and arm. The neurosurgeon referred him to a neurologist who told him that he might have early Parkinsonism, but that he couldn't be certain at this stage. He suggested William return in six months.

During the next several months, William's wife commented that his posture was growing more stooped and that he walked so slowly that she

found herself constantly waiting for him whenever they went out together. The tremor in his hand became a little worse when he was resting,
but went away whenever he used his hand. His wife also complained that
she thought he wasn't paying attention to her since his expression didn't
change no matter what she said.

At the time of William's six-month appointment, the neurologist felt
that he did, indeed, have Parkinsonism. Because the symptoms were becoming severe, he suggested William start on selegiline and then return in
one month to start a second medication if needed. Selegiline helped improve William's walking a bit, and he felt better, but he still had significant
symptoms. The doctor then prescribed levodopa.

William had quite a bit of nausea and some trouble sleeping when he
started the medication, but continued it at his doctor's urging. Within a
few weeks that nausea had disappeared, although he still required a sleeping pill one or two nights a week. He walked and moved normally, however, and his wife said his facial expressions appeared to be increasingly
normal.

William has now been on the medication for three years. He continues
to do quite well, although the doctor has had to increase the dose of medication twice during that time. He has developed an increasingly severe
tremor in his right hand, however, and the tremor has also begun to affect
his left hand. His doctor has told him that he expects William will need an
additional medication to help with his tremor in another year or two.

Surgical Treatment

PALLIDOTOMY AND THALAMOTOMY

The history of surgery for Parkinsonism has been generally disap-
pointing. Before levodopa became available, surgery to cut different

motor tracks in the brain was used to control tremor and abnormal movements. While sometimes successful, the surgery had a very high incidence of complications and severe side effects. These procedures were largely abandoned once levodopa became available.

There has been a resurgence in ablative (meaning to cut) neurosurgery since stereotactic techniques (see chapter 12) have allowed surgeons to accurately make very small cuts in areas deep inside the brain. The theory behind these surgical procedures is simple: since dopamine usually inhibits certain motor tracts in the brain, cutting these tracts could possibly relieve symptoms. Since the tracts in question connect two structures called the globus pallidus and the thalamus, the operations are called either pallidotomy or thalamotomy depending upon which part of the tract is cut.

In general, thalamotomy works best for patients with severe tremor. Thalamotomy reduces tremor on the body side opposite the surgery in up to 90 percent of cases. Pallidotomy seems to help bradykinesia (slowness of movement) more than tremor. Balance and speech may also improve after pallidotomy. Both thalamotomy and pallidotomy also reduce the involuntary movements that occur as a side effect of antiparkinson medicines.

These surgeries definitely have limitations and risks. Thalamotomy is usually performed only on one side of the brain because complication rates are higher and success rates lower when the second side is done. For this reason, the procedures are most appropriate for persons whose Parkinsonism affects one side of their body more than the other. Pallidotomy can be performed on both sides, but it remains unclear how beneficial the second procedure is.

Complications from either surgery can include bleeding within the brain, infection, and unexpected damage to other areas of the brain. Other complications include loss of muscle tone, increased problems with balance, and speech impairment. These are much more likely when patients have surgery on both sides of the brain. It is important to remember that while these surgeries improve symptoms to some degree, medication will still be required and the disease will continue to progress.

TISSUE TRANSPLANTATION

It has always seemed logical that transplanting dopamine-producing tissue into the substantia nigra (the affected part of the brain) would help the symptoms of Parkinsonism. The first surgical attempts to do this involved taking tissue from the patient's own adrenal gland and implanting it into the brain. The procedure was only performed in the U.S. in 1987 and 1988, with less than three hundred patients actually undergoing the surgery. The technique was abandoned because less than 20 percent of patients improved and the complication rate was significant.

Implantation of fetal nerve tissue, which was first performed in Sweden in the late 1980s, has had better success. Theoretically, fetal nerve cells should be able to act in a transplant recipient just the same as in a developing fetus: they grow and establish connections with the nerve cells that lack dopamine connections. Over time the technique has improved as doctors learned what type of fetal cells work best and where they should be placed in the brain.

After the procedure, some of the fetal cells do indeed begin to grow in the host brain. The procedure seems to result in symptom improvement beginning about six months after surgery, with improvement continuing for two to four years. Although patients do seem to improve, none have been able to stop taking medication. The disease also continues to progress despite the transplant.

At this point, fetal cell transplant remains a very experimental procedure performed in only a few centers worldwide. There are, of course, surgical complications that seem similar to those observed with pallidotomy. Additionally, people undergoing the procedure must take immunosuppressive drugs, which can cause additional complications. There are also serious moral and ethical implications involved since the donor tissue must be harvested from aborted human fetuses. Finally, because the procedure is still experimental no insurance company will pay for it.

In summary, current surgical procedures are appropriate only for about 10 percent of Parkinsonism patients. Even those who may benefit from the procedures may not want to take the risks involved if medication is an option. At this time, no type of surgery has any ability to actually reverse the disease; they are simply a way to help control some of its symptoms.

New Developments

Currently, there are a number of techniques and medications being studied in the hope that they will help Parkinsonism patients. Some of the research involves learning more about the function and anatomy of the brain's motor regulating system. Other work investigates possible causes of Parkinsonism in the hope of preventing the disease. The majority of current research (and that most likely to benefit patients who already have the disease) concerns treatment for people who already have Parkinsonism.

The search for more effective medications for Parkinson's disease is likely to be aided by recent research that has concluded there are at least five different brain receptors for dopamine. In the near future, this discovery may allow development of dopamine-like drugs that are more effective and have fewer side effects than those currently available. One such drug, pramipexole (Mirapex®), has recently been released. Although it is not yet clear if pramipexole is truly superior to the other drugs in this class, it seems to prove useful for patients during the early stages of Parkinsonism. A similar medication, ropinirole (Requip®), has recently been released.

Other drugs are being developed that interfere with enzymes that metabolize (break down) dopamine in the body. Several of these drugs, called COMT inhibitors, have either recently been released or are expected to be on the market in the near future. Early results suggest that these drugs are especially effective for patients who have the "wearing off" effect; that is, they get only a few hours relief from each dose of levodopa. One drug in this class, tolcapone (Tasmar®), has been found to cause severe liver damage in some people, however, and is now reserved for patients who do not respond to standard medications. A similar drug, entacapone (Comtess™), should be released by the time this book is printed. Early trials indicate that entacapone does not cause liver damage.

There is also a lot of research geared toward the development of new MAO-B inhibitors similar to selegiline. Hopefully, these drugs will provide further beneficial effects during the early stages of Parkinsonism and may possibly prolong the time until symptoms progress. The drug rasagiline is currently undergoing clinical trials and may be released in the next year or two. Related research is investigating a metabolite of selegiline called des-methyl selegiline. Preliminary research hints that this metabolite may have an effect in slowing the disease.

Surgical research continues in the area of fetal cell transplantation, but other techniques are also being developed. One of these, deep brain stimulation, is already being performed in some centers. Deep brain stimulation involves implanting electrodes into the brain near the location where pallidotomy or thalamotomy would be performed. The electrodes are then connected to a generator similar to a pacemaker and a high-frequency, low-voltage electric current is passed through the electrodes. Early results claim that deep brain stimulation is as effective as surgical procedures without destruction of any brain tissue.

CHAPTER 18

Multiple Sclerosis

What Is Multiple Sclerosis?

Multiple sclerosis (MS) is a chronic disease of the central nervous system. It commonly affects young adults, usually between the ages of twenty and forty. Females are more likely to develop MS than males, and the disease affects Caucasians more frequently than other races.

The major symptom of MS is a sudden loss of neurological function. This loss commonly involves a limited area. For example, sensations may be lost in one area of the body, or weakness can develop in one limb. Usually the symptoms occur in episodes, or attacks, during which new symptoms suddenly develop. Over time, the attacks disturb additional body functions.

MS can behave very differently in different people. About 15 percent of those affected have only occasional problems that subside without long-term disability. In 5 percent of cases the disease progresses rapidly until the person is severely disabled within five or six years. Most cases fall somewhere between these two extremes.

The timeline of the attacks is also variable. Most patients experience a relapsing-remitting course. In relapsing-remitting MS, the patient has a sudden attack that causes one or more neurological problems. Following the attack, the symptoms improve slowly, and the patient does well for months or years, until another attack occurs, usually involving a different area of the body.

A few people have the more severe form of the disease called progressive MS. In progressive MS, the disease steadily causes additional neurological problems. Some people may suffer relapsing-remitting MS for years, and then convert to progressive MS. The exact disease course and specific symptoms that will develop cannot be predicted for any individual case, however.

What Causes Multiple Sclerosis?

CHANGES IN THE BRAIN

MS is referred to as a demyelinating disease. Myelin is a fat and protein membrane that is part of the oligodendrocyte cells, one of the supporting cells of the brain (see chapter 1). The myelin wraps around the axons of nerve cells, enabling them to conduct electrical signals rapidly and efficiently. In some ways, myelin acts like the insulation around a wire. It prevents the nerve's electrical impulses from "shorting out."

Demyelinating diseases such as MS destroy the myelin sheath around axons, presumably by damaging the oligodenrocytes that create and maintain the sheath. When the myelin sheath is injured or destroyed, the axon cannot properly conduct its messages to other nerve cells.

It is believed that MS is an autoimmune disease, that is, a disease in which the immune system attacks part of the body. The immune system of MS patients makes antibodies (substances the immune system makes to attack specific proteins on invading organisms) against the proteins found in myelin. Other cells in their immune system are "sensitized" to myelin proteins, meaning that the immune cells are programmed to attack any cell that has a lot of this protein on their surface.

MS attacks occur in localized areas within the brain causing almost complete destruction of myelin within that small area (or several areas) of the brain. Although the nerve cells and their axons are left intact, with the myelin sheath destroyed they cannot send signals to other nerve cells. The exact area of demyelination determines the symptoms of each attack. If it is in an area carrying motor messages to a part of the body, paralysis occurs in that area. If it is in an area involving one of the senses, that sensation will be at least partially lost.

When the brains of MS patients are examined microscopically, white blood cells are present in the areas of demyelination. These areas can also be detected by an MRI scan, which will indicate localized destruction of white matter in the affected area. The area of demyelination is called a plaque. This finding is not absolutely diagnostic of MS, however, because other conditions that affect the white matter can cause plaques to form.

Who Is Likely to Get Multiple Sclerosis

Although we know that MS is caused by the immune system attacking myelin in the brain, it is not completely clear what causes people to develop the condition. Many hints concerning the causes of MS come from the patterns of the disease. From this information, doctors have evidence that several different factors contribute to developing MS, including genetics environmental factors.

Currently, most doctors believe that only people with certain genetic traits are susceptible to MS onset. Susceptible people must also be exposed to at least one environmental factor (probably a virus) during a certain period of their life to develop the disease. There are several observations that support this theory:

1. Throughout the world, MS is far more common in northern countries than those close to the equator. In the U.S., multiple sclerosis is twice as common in northern states as in southern states.

2. A person's geographic risk is fixed by age fifteen. That is, people who live in the south until age fifteen and then move north will always have the lower southern risk of MS. The opposite effect is true for northerners who move south after age fifteen; they maintain the higher risk.

3. MS is twice as common in women as in men (this is true of many autoimmune diseases).

4. MS is much more common among Caucasians than other races.

5. People with a genetic marker for a certain protein (called HLA-DR2) are much more likely to develop MS.

6. Outbreaks of MS have occurred in certain locations.

7. Having a family history of MS increases the risk of developing MS by up to ten times. Having an identical twin (who has exactly the same genes) with MS increases the risk of developing MS 100 times.

From the above observations, scientists have concluded that exposure to some environmental factor before age fifteen is necessary for a person to eventually develop MS. Throughout the world, this factor is increasingly common the farther one goes from the equator. Because more than two dozen viruses are known to cause a demyelinating disease soon after a person is exposed to them, it seems quite possible that a virus could somehow cause a demyelinating disease to develop years later. It has not yet been definitively proven that any one virus triggers MS, however.

Clearly, there are also genetic factors involved in multiple sclerosis. One current theory is that some people who get MS have a protein in their body that is similar in size and shape to a viral protein (the exact structure of each protein in the body is determined by genes). People with this protein would be at risk of developing an autoimmune disease if they were infected by that virus. People whose genes code for a slightly different protein would not be at risk following infection with the same virus. People who had the protein, but never had the viral infection, would also not develop the disease.

In reality, the development of MS is probably more complex than the circumstances related above. Many researchers believe that several different genes may have to be present for a person to be at risk. It may also be true that more than one viral infection is necessary. There may be other factors involved, but at this time there is no clear evidence as to what those other factors might be. At one time, some people believed that trauma or injury might cause MS, but several studies conducted in the 1990s showed clearly that injury does not cause the disease.

HHV-6

Over the past three years, several scientists have found that Human Herpes Virus-6 (HHV-6), the virus that causes roseola in children, is present in demyelinated areas of MS patients' brains during active attacks. To date, these studies have involved only small numbers of people, and the virus is not found in all people with MS.

There is no proof that HHV-6 actually causes MS since the vast majority of people who have had roseola never develop the disease. It seems possible that the virus is one contributing factor to developing MS, however.

Because of the association between HHV-6 and MS, clinical trials of medications that are effective against this virus have recently been started in a few MS patients. There is currently no evidence that treatment with antiviral drugs will benefit patients with MS, however. It will be several years before the studies are completed.

HEPATITIS B VACCINE

In the mid-1990s, a few people who received the hepatitis B vaccines in France later developed MS. Those affected believed that the vaccine had caused their disease, and the story was picked up throughout the world by the popular press. A study by the French National Drug Surveillance Committee showed clearly that in the twenty million people receiving the vaccine between 1989 and 1997, the frequency of MS was actually *lower* than in the general population. Similar results have been reported from Australia, Canada, Germany, the U.K. and the U.S.

Unfortunately, the studies done by these governments never received as much attention as the original "scare" stories did, leading many people to still believe that the hepatitis B vaccine might cause MS. Hepatitis B infects four million people each year and about 25 percent of those infected will die of the disease. No one should refuse a hepatitis B vaccine for fear of developing MS.

What Are the Symptoms of Multiple Sclerosis?

The exact symptoms caused by MS are different in every person because the areas of the brain involved in the demyelination are different in each case. Almost any symptom that could be caused by a stroke can occur in MS. Usually, the symptoms caused by any one attack do not involve large areas of the body. Paralysis or loss of sensation of both legs can occur if MS affects the spinal cord, however.

Problems with vision are very common and can include partial blindness, double vision, and difficulty focusing the eyes. Optic neuritis, an inflammation of the nerve connecting the eye with the brain, is one of the common symptoms of MS. Any vision changes should be treated right away or permanent blindness can result.

Weakness, numbness, and spasticity can occur almost anywhere in the body. Abnormal sensations, such as "pins and needles" or burning pain, are also frequent. Difficulties with bladder and bowel functions are common, and impotence or other sexual problems may occur. Emotional and thinking problems can also occur.

Some of the primary neurological problems caused by MS can result in other, secondary problems. For example, inability to empty the bladder completely may cause repeated urinary tract infections. If muscle function is abnormal in one shoulder, muscle imbalances can affect posture or even walking. Inactivity can lead to other muscle weakness, osteoporosis, and chronic pain.

The most important aspect of MS is not any single symptom, however: it is the way the disease acts over time. MS is described as a progressive, intermittent, and relapsing disease. This means that over the very long term (many years) patients will invariably get worse. Over the shorter term, however, it is characterized by acute attacks during which new symptoms develop, followed by recovery, during which the new symptom partially resolves. Following recovery there may be no new symptoms for years until another attack occurs.

A few patients (less than 5 percent) do not follow the normal intermittent course of MS but rather have progressive MS. These patients do not have attack and recovery phases, but instead experience a slow, steady progression of their disease. About half of MS patients who initially have the intermittent form of the disease will develop the progressive form after ten years. In either case, people with progressive MS tend to worsen much more rapidly than those with the intermittent form. On average, about five years will pass between the onset of progressive MS and total disability.

Unlike most other diseases, MS patients usually have more symptoms during warm weather or if they become overheated. It is uncertain if heat actually worsens the disease or if it simply makes the symptoms more apparent. Pregnancy seems to reduce the chance of an attack. The benefit of pregnancy is temporary, however. During the first three months after birth, the chance of having an attack increases by more than 70 percent.

Diagnosis of Multiple Sclerosis

Doctors make the diagnosis of MS based on what are called clinical criteria. This means there is no test that indicates with certainty if a patient has the disease. Rather, when doctors suspect a patient has MS they must monitor the patient's symptoms over time. Once a patient exhibits certain symptoms in a pattern, doctors can decide that the patient has MS. At the same time, doctors must be sure that no other disease is present that could mimic the symptoms of MS.

The first step is to insure that the patient is suffering from a demyelinating disease. Demyelinating areas of the brain and spinal cord (plaques) can usually be detected by an MRI scan. While plaques are strong evidence of MS, by themselves they are not diagnostic of the disease because they can occur in other diseases. On the other hand, a normal MRI scan does not absolutely rule out a diagnosis of MS either, since 5 percent of MS patients will have a normal MRI scan during the disease's early phases. Evoked potentials (see chapter 4) may show demyelination in those cases where the MRI scan is normal. Evoked potential can also provide evidence of scarring along nerve pathways, especially involving the optic nerve and spinal cord, that is not apparent on a neurological exam.

The second criteria needed for diagnosing MS is that the patient must have either two separate episodes of neurologic problems at least one month apart or that the disease has shown a progressive course over six months. Given these criteria, a person obviously cannot be diagnosed as having MS upon onset of symptoms. The disease may be suspected after a single episode or attack, but cannot be diagnosed until another episode happens, which could be years later.

When the diagnosis of MS is in question, the doctor may order other tests. These will not actually prove that the patient has MS, but can eliminate other possibilities or may provide further evidence suggesting that MS is indeed the problem. Usually, cerebrospinal fluid will be obtained by a spinal tap and tested for certain immune system proteins that can indicate an autoimmune disease is present. About 90 percent of MS patients will have elevated levels of an antibody (one of the immune proteins) called IgG in their spinal fluid. These proteins form a band, called an oligoclonal band, on a certain test. While oligoclonic bands are associated with MS, they also occur in other diseases and are not always present in MS patients.

Sometimes the diagnosis of MS can be made easily and quickly. Other people may suffer vague or unusual complaints for several years before the diagnosis is confirmed, or even suspected. Unfortunately, when a long time passes between the first symptoms and making the diagnosis, patients may be told they are "hysterical" or suffering from stress and depression.

The Course and Outcome of Multiple Sclerosis

When a person is diagnosed as having MS their first question is usually, "What is going to happen?" Unfortunately, it is difficult to predict the course of MS in any individual. Research has shown, however, that how the disease acts over the first five years will often predict how it will act for the rest of the patient's life.

In most cases, MS follows one of four clinical courses:

1. A benign sensory form, in which the attacks are characterized by loss of sensations or visual symptoms, but not weakness or paralysis. People with this form of MS usually do not develop severe long-term disability.
2. A relapsing-remitting form, characterized by partial or total recovery after attacks involving both sensory and muscle problems. This is the most common type of MS.
3. A progressive form that continues to steadily worsen with very little recovery between attacks. This is the rarest and severest form of MS. Most people with this form will become severely disabled within five years.

4. A relapsing-remitting course that later becomes steadily progressive, called secondary progressive MS. This eventually occurs in almost half of the people who originally had a
   relapsing-remitting course.

Those who have mostly sensory symptoms, such as numbness,
tingling, and vision problems, during their early attacks generally do
better over the long term than other patients. Those who have mostly
motor symptoms, including weakness, tremor, and incoordination,
usually have a more severe and progressive course. Although severe
disability can be caused by MS, it does not lower the life expectancy
of its victims.

Treatment of Multiple Sclerosis

The treatment of MS must take place on several levels. First, there are
drugs taken on a regular basis, including some very new medications
that may slow progression of the disease. The second type is taken during an acute attack in an attempt to lessen its severity. Finally, medications and other treatments are used to help reduce the symptoms from
demyelinating attacks that have already occurred.

TREATMENTS TO SLOW THE DISEASE COURSE

Interferon Beta

Interferon beta (Betaseron®, Betaferon®) has been available since
1994. The drug is similar to the chemical interferon that is produced
by the human immune system. In the body, interferon reduces the immune system's responses to certain stimulations. Theoretically, Interferon beta could reduce the immune system's attacks on myelin in
people with MS.

In clinical studies, Interferon beta does appear to reduce the frequency and severity of attacks in about two-thirds of people with
recurrent-relapsing MS. Attacks were less frequent in people taking

the medication. When attacks did occur, they were generally less severe. Further, over time people taking Interferon beta had fewer new plaques observed on an MRI scan than those who were not taking the drug. Patients have only been studied for a few years, however, so it is not clear if the effects will wear off over time.

Interferon beta is currently approved only for recurrent-relapsing MS. However, in late 1998, a large European trial (718 patients) of Interferon beta (Betaseron) for treatment of secondary progressive MS was stopped early because the drug clearly slowed the disease. In this study, the drug slowed progression of disability by nine to twelve months and reduced the number of attacks by over 30 percent.

A separate clinical trial of Betaseron for secondary progressive MS in the U.S. and Canada is already well underway and results are expected within two years. Although Betaseron is not yet officially approved in the U.S. for use in progressive MS, doctors can prescribe it for this purpose.

Interferon beta can only be administered by injection and must be injected every other day in order to be effective. The medication must also be kept refrigerated at all times. Interferon beta commonly causes some side effects, although they do not usually prove severe. Most people will experience flu-like symptoms for at least the first few weeks. The drug also causes reactions (swelling, redness, discoloration, pain) at the injection sites. There have been a few reports of severe depression in people taking Interferon beta, and it is believed to cause birth defects if taken during pregnancy.

Interferon Alpha

Interferon alpha (Avonex™) is chemically different from Interferon beta, being chemically more similar to natural human interferon. It also has the advantage of only requiring injection once a week instead of every other day as does Interferon beta.

Along with Interferon beta, Interferon alpha was shown to reduce the number and severity of attacks in people with recurrent-relapsing

MS. Because this drug was only released in 1997, it is not as well documented as Interferon beta, and it may not work quite as well as Interferon beta does. At the very least, however, it offers an alternative to Interferon beta for patients unable to tolerate that medication.

Recent studies hint that Interferon alpha may be as effective, if not more effective, than Interferon beta, however. Results from a large (560 patients), multicenter clinical study of Interferon alpha conducted in Europe, Australia, and Canada were released in late 1998. The study followed patients for two years and found about a 30 percent reduction in the rate of MS attacks for those patients taking Interferon alpha. Many patients taking the drug had no attacks during the study period, and the severity of attacks that did occur was reduced. The number of plaques detected by MRI scan was significantly reduced in almost all patients taking the drug. In this study, however, the doses of Interferon alpha used were higher than the doses approved by the FDA.

Interferon alpha causes flu-like symptoms in most people during the first few weeks of treatment, and also may cause birth defects. It does not appear to cause severe depression, however, and does not seem to cause as much irritation at the injection site as Interferon beta does.

An oral form of Interferon alpha has been developed and is currently undergoing testing in animals. It will be several years before the oral form might possibly be released for human use, however.

Glatamier Acetate

Glatamier acetate, also called copolymer 1 (Copaxone®), is a synthetic protein resembling the myelin protein that is the focus of the autoimmune reaction in MS. Glatamier seems to block this reaction to some degree and lessens the severity of the autoimmune reaction. The drug has been available for just eighteen months, but early studies suggest it lessens the frequency of attacks in people who have the recurrent-relapsing form of MS. It may not be as effective as the interferons, but it does provide an alternative for people who can't tolerate the side effects of those medications.

Glatamier must be given by injection every day. Local irritation, redness, and itching at the injection site are common. It can also cause weight gain, increased fatigue, and muscle weakness. A few people experience breathing difficulties or chest pain after taking it, and others report dizziness or flushing. The medication also causes allergies in a significant number of people, may trigger migraine headaches, cause swelling of the hands and feet, and has been reported to cause sexual problems in males.

Immunosuppressive Medications

When people with the more severe, progressive form of MS don't respond to one of the above medications, they may require a trial of immunosuppressive medications. These medications are taken by organ transplant recipients and used to treat some types of cancer. All of them suppress the entire immune system, which may (or may not) help the disease, but sometimes presents the only hope available for severe cases. Closporine, cyclophosphamide, methotrexate, and azothiprine are all immunosuppressants that have been used to treat MS. All these medications can cause a severe drop in white blood cell counts making the patient very susceptible to infection. They may also cause sterility and cancer and are therefore used only in the most severe cases of MS. To date, there have not been any studies demonstrating whether these agents are clearly effective in progressive MS, but several studies suggest they do benefit at least some patients.

Two immunosuppressing drugs appear to show particular promise for treating MS. The first, cladribine, is currently being studied for use in treating MS. In a recent study, patients with chronic progressive MS who took a four-month course of cladribine improved for at least eighteen months. They also had improvement in the number of plaques seen on an MRI scan. Some small studies have also reported that cladribine has a similar effect in patients with remitting-relapsing MS.

Another immune suppressing drug, mitoxantrone (Novantrone®) holds perhaps even more promise because it kills the specific types of white blood cells that are active in MS. In the U.S., mitoxantrone is currently approved for treating certain forms of adult leukemia and advanced prostate cancer. In other countries, it is also used to treat lymphoma, breast cancer, and hepatoma.

A few small trials have studied mitoxantrone as a treatment for progressive forms of MS and demonstrated that it has some benefit. The studies were not large enough to draw definite conclusions, however. A larger study of almost 200 patients followed for two years was completed in late 1998. This study documented that patients receiving mitoxantrone had fewer attacks, slower onset of disability, and were far less likely to develop new abnormalities on their MRI scans. The drug appeared to be effective for patients with both the intermittent-relapsing form of MS and those with the progressive form.

Mitoxantrone has to be given by intravenous infusion so it must be administered in a doctor's office or hospital outpatient facility. It only has to be given once every few months to be effective, however. Unfortunately, the drug has several significant side effects. Extended use of the medication can lead to significant heart problems in certain people, and it is possible that the long-term use required for treating MS might make this complication more frequent. It is also uncertain if the drug might interact with other medications used to treat MS.

The FDA is analyzing results from clinical trials to determine if there is sufficient evidence to approve mitoxantrone for use in MS. In all likelihood, however, they will request further clinical trials to decide its long-term safety, a process that could take several years.

TREATMENTS FOR ACUTE ATTACKS OF MULTIPLE SCLEROSIS

Cortisones

The corticosteroids (cortisone-like medicines) are used to relieve inflammation (swelling caused by an immune reaction or tissue damage) in different parts of the body. During an acute MS attack, these drugs can reduce the amount of inflammation in the brain caused by the autoimmune attack against myelin.

Most neurologists believe that giving a high dose of corticosteroids at the beginning of an MS attack will shorten the attack's length and limit its severity. Treatment usually begins with a high dose of corticosteroids given intravenously over four days, and then a tapered dose is continued by mouth for two to four weeks. Any of several different corticosteroids may be used, including dexamethasone, prednisone, betamethasone, or prednisolone.

Corticosteroids have several side effects. The drugs interfere with the body's ability to fight infection, so people taking these medications should avoid contact with anyone who has a contagious infection. The medications also increase appetite and cause fluid retention, resulting in some weight gain. They can interfere with the body's ability to metabolize sugar, thereby worsening diabetes. The drugs can also cause birth defects and will pass into a mother's breast milk. Finally, some people will develop heartburn or gastritis while taking corticosteroids, especially when taken by mouth.

Corticosteroids can cause mood changes, including euphoria, depression, anxiety, and sleeplessness. These mood alterations may be quite mild or can be very severe. Mood alterations are quite unpredictable. A person who has previously had no emotional effects from taking corticosteroids may develop severe emotional changes the next time they require the medication. Further, people with a history of mood disorders or anxiety are more likely to have emotional difficulties.

Anyone who requires frequent doses of corticosteroids over a long period of time may develop permanent swelling of the face (called a "moon-shaped" face), elevated blood pressure, easy bruising of the skin, or menstrual irregularities. Long-term use can also cause osteoporosis (thinning of the bones), and in particular may cause problems with the hip joints.

When patients receive a high dose of corticosteroids to stop an MS attack, their body stops producing its own cortisone. This is the reason the doctor will slowly taper the medication; it is extremely important not to stop taking them abruptly. Severe effects, including low blood sugar, low blood pressure, heart failure, and kidney problems can result.

Despite their side effects, corticosteroids do shorten acute attacks and make the victim increasingly likely to recover function following the attack. Most doctors do not recommend treating every single attack, however, reserving the medications for severe attacks involving vision, paralysis, or several problems occurring together.

Some doctors also use corticosteroids to treat progressive MS. In these cases, the medications are generally given as a single large dose once a month. When only a single high dose is given, the body continues to manufacture its own cortisone, so tapering it is not necessary.

TREATING THE SYMPTOMS OF MULTIPLE SCLEROSIS

Numbness and Tingling

Numbness means being unable to feel sensations from a part of the body. Tingling is the feeling you experience when your foot falls asleep. Tingling is usually temporary in MS, signalling either the beginning of an attack that will progress to numbness, or occurring as a previously numb area begins to heal. It can be quite aggravating if it lasts for a long time.

Numbness may be total (no sensations) or partial (sensing a touch, but not being able to tell the difference between hot and cold, for example). Often the numb area functions just fine: a numb hand can grip and perform all its normal tasks, for example, although it will be clumsy because of the lack of sensation.

There are no effective medical treatments for numbness, but there are several medications that may help the tingling "pins and needles" sensations. Antiseizure medications such as gabapentin (Neurontin) or carbamazepine (Tegretol) often reduce the severity of tingling. Certain antidepressants, particularly amitriptyline (Elavil), may also be effective, especially if the sensations are worse at night.

Problems with walking and balance may be caused by a variety of factors present in MS. Demyelination affecting the coordination or balance centers of the brain can obviously cause such problems, as can muscle weakness in the legs and hips. Demyelination in the spinal cord generally causes severe difficulty in walking and may require the use of a walker or wheelchair. No medications can help either walking or balance disturbances.

Tremors

Tremors (uncontrollable shaking) occur when the demyelination of MS affects an area of the brain that controls muscle function. Usually these take the form of intention tremors, which are tremors that occur only when the affected limb is performing some activity. The hands are most often affected, and tremors can range from very mild to shaking so severe that the limb is almost useless.

There are some medications that help control tremors, but none are completely effective. The medications used to treat the tremors of Parkinsonism are generally not effective for the tremors of MS. Medications that block the effects of adrenaline, such as propranolol (Inderal®), and antiseizure medications are sometimes effective. Tranquilizers such as alprazolam (Xanax) may also be effective.

Muscle Spasms

A lot of the pain experienced by MS patients involves the muscles. Muscle spasms can occur anywhere in the body, although the legs and back are affected most frequently. Spasms may occur with overexertion, but can also begin spontaneously, especially at night. Sudden episodes of muscle spasms cause an extremely painful, cramping pain, while mild, chronic muscle spasms can cause a deep aching pain.

Baclofen is usually the first medication used for both chronic spasms and episodes of severe spasm. The medication is taken orally three or four times a day and reduces or eliminates spasms in over half of all cases. Baclofen may cause sedation, mild muscle weakness, or dry mouth, but otherwise has few side effects. A few people respond better to standard muscle relaxers such as cyclobenzaprine (Flexeril®) or Valium than they do to baclofen, and in severe cases more than one drug may be required.

A newer medication, tizanidine, has recently been released in the U.S. after being used in Europe for several years. Tizanidine seems as effective as baclofen overall, but it may work in some cases where baclofen was not effective. It also causes less muscle weakness than baclofen, although it is more sedating.

People who have permanent spasticity from MS paralysis, or extreme episodes of muscle spasms that don't respond to oral medications, may be candidates for an implanted baclofen pump. This device is surgically implanted under the skin and contains its own battery supply and drug reservoir. It delivers baclofen directly to the cerebrospinal fluid surrounding the spinal cord. It may prove dramatically effective—even when all standard medications have failed.

If the spasms are localized to one or two muscle groups, injections of botulinum toxin (Botox®) may be performed. The injection will usually stop contraction in the affected muscle. Each injection may last weeks or months, meaning that it can stop spasm until an acute attack has passed. Unfortunately, the treatments are quite expensive and are not covered by all insurance plans.

Aching in the back, legs, or arms is quite common in MS patients. It is usually caused by a low-grade spasm in the muscles of the spine and trunk. This may be especially severe with prolonged standing or walking, or it may be most severe during nighttime after an active day. Muscle relaxants and anti-inflammatory medications, such as Motrin, are usually helpful.

Pain

There are many different causes of pain in MS. Demyelination of nerves can itself cause pain, which is usually felt as an intense burning or stinging sensation. One form this pain may take in MS patients is trigeminal neuralgia, an extremely painful condition involving the face and jaw. Demyelination in the spinal cord can cause a stinging pain that radiates from the back to the legs or arms.

The chronic burning pain of demyelination can usually be effectively treated with anticonvulsant medications. Gabapentin (Neurontin), carbamazepine (Tegretol), and valproate (Depakote) are usually effective. It may take several weeks of treatment, however, before the medications begin to work. These medications all cause sedation, but it usually disappears after a few weeks of treatment. The tricyclic antidepressants, particularly amitriptyline (Elavil), can also help reduce demyelination pain. Standard narcotic pain medications are usually not very effective against this type of pain, however.

Trigeminal neuralgia is treated using the same medications for demyelination pain. When they are not effective, surgery or radiation treatment of the trigeminal nerve may be necessary to stop pain. These latter procedures will cause permanent numbness of the face, however, and should only be employed in cases where no medical therapy has worked.

Bladder, Urinary, and Sexual Problems

At least 80 percent of MS patients have some difficulty with their urinary system. MS can interfere with the transmission of nerve signals to the bladder and urinary sphincter (the muscle at the bladder opening that holds in urine). If the bladder muscles are unable to relax, a spastic bladder that can't hold much urine results. If bladder muscles become paralyzed, the bladder is unable to empty properly. If the sphincter muscle becomes spastic, the bladder may not empty at all, while if it is weakened, urine will leak out at unexpected times.

Common symptoms of bladder problems may include the need to urinate frequently, difficulty in starting urination, waking up several times at night to urinate, or incontinence (the inability to hold in urine). Left untreated, bladder problems can result in repeated infections or even kidney damage. Obviously, they can also cause social embarrassment. Most bladder difficulties in MS patients can be treated effectively with medications, but some people will eventually require catheterization (inserting a soft rubber tube into the bladder to drain urine). Any MS sufferer who has bladder problems should see a urologist for a complete bladder evaluation.

Bladder spasms and a spastic bladder can usually be treated with medications called anticholinergics. Propantheline and oxybutynin are two of the most commonly used anticholinergics. They will usually improve bladder symptoms, but can cause dry mouth and unpleasant side effects in some people. Terazosin, a different type of medication, can be an effective alternative for people who can't tolerate anticholinergic medicines.

Those who find that they have to get up frequently during the night because of a full bladder may benefit from desmopressin. This medication, taken as a nasal spray at bedtime, is actually a synthetic form of the body's own hormone that reduces urine production. It has few side effects and can prove dramatically effective. It may be contraindicated in people who have heart failure, however.

Male impotence, and lack of lubrication or vaginal numbness in females, sometimes occurs in people with MS. Viagra® is an effective treatment for most male MS patients with impotence. In the few cases when Viagra is not effective, Caverject®, which must be injected near the base of the penis, will usually create an erection. Lack of lubrication is easily resolved with any of dozens of vaginal lubricants available.

Alteration of sexual drive is actually more common than physical sexual problems. Although certain brain lesions can directly alter sexual drive, depression is a much more frequent cause of sexual disinterest in MS patients than brain damage. Often the newer antidepressants, known as selective serotonin reuptake inhibitors, or SSRIs, can rapidly treat depression and restore sexual interest.

Bowel Problems
Bowel incontinence (inability to control bowel movements) is rare in MS, but constipation does occur frequently. Diarrhea, or diarrhea al-

ternating with constipation, can also occur. While bowel problems can be caused by the disease itself, often the problems are the result of inactivity, poor diet caused by eating difficulties or depression, or the side effects of medications.

Most MS patients can avoid bowel problems if they drink enough fluids (at least six to eight glasses daily), take fiber supplements, and use stool softeners such as mineral oil. Enemas or laxatives may be used in moderation, but using them every day will often worsen bowel problems over the long term.

Thinking and Memory Problems

Between 40 and 60 percent of people with MS have some cognitive problems (meaning difficulty with thinking or memory). Of all the different problems the disease causes, this is perhaps the most terrifying. Patients may be afraid that they will become unable to work or even incompetent to manage their own legal and financial affairs. Because of the fear they cause, cognitive problems are often ignored or denied by the MS sufferer.

Problems with attention and concentration are the most commonly reported types of cognitive difficulty. For example, someone may have difficulty returning to a task if he or she is interrupted, or may be unable to maintain concentration long enough to finish a complicated task such as writing a letter. Many MS sufferers also notice it is more difficult, and takes longer, for them to learn new material. They may also have problems making quick decisions, often finding that after they have made a hasty decision, they later realize it was incorrect. A few people with MS have some trouble organizing and setting priorities or controlling their expression of emotions.

Memory is the intellectual function most commonly affected by MS. Short-term memory ("Where did I put that?" memory) is often affected, but some specific memories may also be altered. For example, an MS patient may suddenly find they have difficulty remembering the names of cooking utensils, although they know exactly when and how to use them. Many people with MS experience occasional difficulty finding the right word, or putting words together quickly to say exactly what they mean. This difficulty appears to be more of a memory problem than a speech or thinking problem.

Reasoning, problem solving, and judgment are probably the least affected mental functions. MS patients rarely have problems with reasoning, making appropriate decisions, or other purely intellectual functions. IQ scores, for example, are not affected in MS patients unless the test used is one that scores speed heavily. MS patients do find that they make mistakes when they are rushed or distracted, but when they are not hurried, they are just as intelligent as ever. Just the same as physical problems, mental problems will lessen after an acute flare up of the condition.

It's important to remember that people can compensate for memory and thinking problems just as they can for physical problems. Of course, keeping lists and calendars is the best way to overcome short-term memory problems. Concentration and attention problems will be minimized if arrangements are made so that the person can focus on one project at a time. This may be as simple as letting people around them know not to interrupt when they are working or using do-not-disturb signs and telephone answering machines more frequently. It may also involve scheduling work and home activities so that they can be completed in order, one at a time. Mistakes in judgment will occur less frequently if decisions are not rushed. Taking a few minutes to think through a decision may help avoid errors.

Fatigue and Depression

Most MS patients say that fatigue is their most troublesome symptom, particularly during the late phases of the disease. Fatigue seems particularly bad during the hot summer months. Most MS patients find they must plan to rest or nap during the day in order to function well in the evening. Some medications may also help fatigue symptoms. Amantadine (Symmetrel), a medication originally used to prevent influenza, appears to reduce fatigue in MS, although no one is sure how it works. Amantadine does have some side effects including dry mouth, blurred vision, and constipation. Pemoline and methylphenidate (Ritalin) may also be effective, but can prove habit forming.

Many MS patients also experience depression during their illness, and a few develop emotional outbursts. These symptoms may be caused by demyelination in the frontal lobes, as a side effect of medications, or simply because of MS. In any case, antidepressant medications are usually quite effective. Of the antidepressants, Imipramine (Tofranil®) appears particularly effective for mood swings. Paxil™ may prove more effective for those patients who have depression and burning pain from demyelination.

OTHER TREATMENTS

Physical Therapy and Exercise

The relapsing and remitting course of MS means that people will have different physical problems at different times. Physical therapy is invaluable in maintaining as much function as possible during acute attacks and restoring function once the attack has resolved.

When acute episodes cause paralysis of part of the body, physical therapy is used to prevent contractures (permanent shortening of the muscles) and to reduce the amount of muscle spasm. During the worst part of an attack, physical therapy may be needed on a daily basis. Treatments such as electrical muscle stimulation can also help to maintain muscle strength during these episodes so that rehabilitation will be easier once the attack has passed.

When an attack has resolved, physical therapy is used to retrain muscles to function properly. This may be as simple as a general conditioning and strengthening program, or as complicated as learning how to walk again. Physical therapy is particularly helpful for those patients having problems with walking, balance, and endurance. It can also be invaluable for people experiencing a lot of muscle spasms.

Regular exercise helps minimize many of the symptoms of MS. Patients who participate in an aerobic exercise program have better bladder and bowel function, less fatigue and depression, and an increase in participation in social activities at every stage of the disease. MS patients who don't exercise are far more likely to suffer loss of trunk control, shortening and weakness of leg muscles, inefficient breathing with a higher risk of pneumonia, and osteoporosis.

The exercise program must be designed for the capabilities of each MS patient and then adjusted as their symptoms change. An experienced physical therapist is probably the best person to design such a program, but personal trainers who have experience working with disabled people can also create an effective program, and often at lower cost.

While physical therapy and exercise are of great benefit, it is important to remember that overheating can make MS symptoms worse. Exercise should be done in a cool environment with alternating periods of exercise and rest to prevent overheating.

Occupational Therapy

Occupational therapy works together with physical therapy for problems involving walking, standing, and the use of arms and hands. Occupational therapy focuses on ways to accomplish specific, everyday tasks while physical therapy focuses on restoring muscle strength and motion.

Occupational therapists often fit braces or sprints and provide aids such as canes or walkers. They also supply special devices to assist in performing everyday activities such as washing, using the toilet, dressing, driving, and housekeeping. Finally, occupational therapists are active in retraining hand-eye coordination and manual dexterity. This often includes exercises for fingers and hands specifically tailored to an individual's level of functioning.

Occupational therapists will often visit the house or workplace and give advice concerning modifications that can help an individual's specific needs. A number of useful devices are available such as button hooks, rocker knives, pot and pan stabilizers, and special grips for pens and pencils.

ALTERNATIVE MEDICINE AND
MULTIPLE SCLEROSIS

MS can be a devastating disease, but it is one for which much research is conducted. More than most neurological diseases, MS patients tend to be very involved with their own treatment, and many spend a lot of time investigating new treatments and medications for their disease. At the same time, many alternative or nonmedical therapists are attempting to treat MS.

Alternative therapies may include drugs (remember, many of today's medications are simply purified herbal remedies), diets, food supplements, mental and physical exercises, and lifestyle regimens. Acupuncture, relaxation techniques, chiropractic, yoga, hypnosis, biofeedback, aromatherapy, homeopathy, reflexology, hypnotherapy, naturopathy, and various schools of massage are also considered alternative therapies.

Obviously there is nothing wrong with trying alternative therapies. Medicine cannot offer a cure and can only slow the disease and offer supportive care. However, keep in mind that medical treatment *can* slow the disease and offer supportive care. Adding an alternative therapy to your medical regimen may help and will rarely cause harm. Stopping your medical therapy to try an alternative treatment may allow the disease to progress more rapidly.

Understandably, people who suffer from MS are often desperate. Very often they are young people who suddenly find they have an incurable disease that has a major effect on their life. Because alternative treatments are not regulated by the FDA or other government agencies, there are plenty of unscrupulous people who will attempt to take advantage of a desperate MS patient. While there are honest and honorable people who offer alternative medical treatments, there are also greedy charlatans who will take advantage of an MS sufferer's desperation.

By definition, alternative therapies have not been scientifically documented as effective against any specific diseases or conditions.

As a rule, they do not fit with current scientific knowledge about the cause of a particular disease such as MS. That doesn't mean they don't work. Several alternative therapies of twenty years ago are now part of mainstream medicine.

Generally most people, including doctors, feel that if the treatment appears harmless, it's worth a try. Remember, however, that because alternative treatments are not held to medical standards, their advocates (or salesman) can make almost any claim they wish. For a medication to be approved for public use, it must first be proven in scientific studies as both safe and effective. For an herbal treatment or any other form of alternative medicine to be approved for public consumption—well actually, it just gets put on the market. If I pull out the grass in my backyard and claim it's an ancient Chinese cure for cancer, I can try to sell it. In fact, the government has to prove it does not work, or is not safe, to stop me from selling it.

And this does happen. Just because a product is "natural" doesn't mean it's safe. Rabies virus is completely natural. So is cyanide (easily extracted from almond shells and peach pits). In fact, over two hundred "completely natural" products of one type or another have been found to be dangerous and removed from public consumption over the last decade.

Just because a certain therapy is recommended by a medical doctor—only one medical doctor—doesn't mean it's safe and effective. Scientifically well-researched medical treatments are published in reputable medical journals where every doctor can read about them and use them. Any doctor whose treatment is "ignored" by the medical community hasn't proven (to anyone of reputable standing) that it works.

Again, I've no objection to alternative medicine and have no doubt it contains many beneficial treatments. Chapter sixteen, for example, covers two alternative medicines (ginkgo and carnitine) right alongside those developed by the drug companies. Be careful, however. If a treatment is extremely expensive, contains any "secret" ingredients, or is available only by mail order, be suspicious. If a treatment really worked for everyone who tried it, it wouldn't be a secret.

Avoid "testimonials" from "satisfied customers," especially when only first names or initials are used. MS is a disease of relapses and remissions. If a lot of people with MS drink magic spring water during an attack, most will be better three months later, and they'll all be willing to write a testimonial. Of course, if a lot of people with MS don't drink magic spring water during an attack, most will be better three months later, too.

The National Multiple Sclerosis Society's Information Resource Center (see appendix F) monitors alternative therapies for both effectiveness and fraudulent claims. They can provide objective information about any therapy you are considering.

CASE STUDY: Multiple Sclerosis

When she was twenty-six years old, Nancy, had a sudden episode of severely blurred vision in her right eye. She saw an eye doctor who found nothing wrong with the eye itself and referred her to a neurologist. An MRI scan of her brain was normal, and by the time she'd returned to see the neurologist a second time, her vision had almost returned to normal. She was scheduled for a follow-up appointment in six months, but since she was feeling fine, she canceled it.

About a year later, Nancy experienced a burning pain and tingling in her left leg. Again she was evaluated by the neurologist who found nothing wrong. He suggested she might be under a lot of stress and recommended she see a psychologist. Three months later, she had a similar episode involving her right arm. After a week she returned to the neurologist who repeated her MRI scan.

This time the scan revealed plaques, areas of demyelination (loss of the normal character of the white matter) in her brain. After seeing her scan, the neurologist suspected Nancy had MS and performed a spinal tap. The cerebrospinal fluid showed the characteristic protein bands that are often found in MS.

Because all her episodes had involved sensation problems, the neurologist felt that Nancy probably had benign sensory MS, a form of the disease that usually doesn't progress to severe disability. He recommended that Nancy not begin any of the more potent medications to prevent MS attacks because the risk of side effects was probably greater than the risk of having future attacks that might cause major problems. He would prefer that Nancy contact him immediately at the start of her next attack and receive cortisone treatments.

Nancy asked for a second opinion from another neurologist, who was in complete agreement. Over the following three years, Nancy has had two more attacks. She has received cortisone treatments both times, first at an outpatient chemotherapy center and then orally. Both attacks ended within days. She continued to have burning pain in her leg and arm, but the neurologist placed her on an antiseizure medication, which has almost eliminated the pain.

Although Nancy has done very well to date, her neurologist has cautioned her that it is possible her MS could become more severe or progressive. If this happens, she will probably begin taking one of the interferon medications. It is also quite possible, however, that her disease will continue in its benign form.

Glossary

Acuity: clarity or distinctness of hearing or sight.

Agnosia: loss of the ability to recognize objects, people, sounds, shapes, or smells. Usually occurs with problems involving the parietal lobe of the cerebral hemispheres.

Agraphia: loss of ability to write.

Angioplasty: a procedure to restore the opening of an artery, usually by threading a balloon-tipped catheter to the site of blockage and then inflating the balloon to compress plaque back against the wall of the artery.

Aneurysm: a balloonlike, weakened outpouching of an arterial wall. Aneurysms can rupture causing severe bleeding.

Anosmia: loss of sense of smell.

Aphasia: loss of the ability to speak or write, or of the ability to understand speech or written words.

Apraxia: inability to plan and perform purposeful movements while still having the ability to move.

Ataxia: walking that is clumsy or uncoordinated.

Arachnoid mater: thin layer pressed against inner surface of the dura mater by cerebrospinal fluid pressure. This layer has a spiderweb-like appearance.

Arteriography: an x-ray of the arteries, performed by directly injecting x-ray dye into the arteries themselves.

Arteriovenous malformations: a tangled mass of abnormal arteries and veins.

Atherosclerosis: disease of the arteries characterized by fatty deposits in the wall of an artery that eventually become large enough to significantly obstruct blood flow through the artery. These areas can also serve as a focus to cause blood clots (thrombus) within the artery.

Basilar artery: the central artery of the brain stem, formed when two vertebral arteries join together.

Blood–brain barrier: a protective barrier around the blood vessels of the brain that prevents some substances from entering brain tissue.

Brain stem: comprises midbrain, pons, and medulla oblongata, as well as the cerebellum.

Carotid endarterectomy: a surgical procedure to remove plaque from the inside of the carotid artery.

Cerebellum: largest part of the brain stem, it sits under the cerebral hemispheres and is connected to the pons. Important for coordination of movement.

Cerebral cortex: the outside layer of the cerebrum, made up of gray matter (nerve cell bodies).

Cerebral edema: swelling of the brain and brain's cells.

Cerebral hemisphere: one of the large paired structures making up the largest and most complex part of the brain. It has four lobes: frontal, temporal, parietal, and occipital.

Cerebral infarction: death of the cells in a part of the brain.

Cerebral hemorrhage: bleeding into the brain itself. Sometimes used to refer to bleeding inside the skull but outside the brain. See *Subarachnoid hemorrhage*.

Cerebrospinal fluid: the fluid that bathes the brain and spinal cord.

Cerebrum: the largest area of the brain, composed of the two cerebral hemispheres.

Cerebrovascular disease: any disease involving the blood vessels of the brain usually meaning atherosclerosis of the brain's arteries.

Choroid plexus: vascular areas in the ventricles that produce cerebrospinal fluid.

Concussion: unconsciousness after a head injury.

Congenital: existing before or at birth.

Contrecoup: bruising of the brain tissue in the side opposite to where the blow was struck, caused by the brain "bouncing" within the skull.

Contracture: permanent shortening of the muscles, fixing one or more joints in a flexed (bent) position. Contracture can occur after a stroke or other neurologic disease causes paralysis in a limb.

Corpus callosum: the large bundles of white matter (fibers) connecting the two cerebral hemispheres.

Craniotomy: surgery that removes a portion of the skull to gain access to the brain.

Dementia: severe deterioration of mental function. The affected person loses the ability to function in reality.

Diabetes insipidus: abnormal secretion of the water-balancing hormones of the brain causing large volumes of urine to be produced, resulting in dehydration.

Diffuse axonal injury (DAI): widespread tearing of nerve fibers throughout the brain usually caused by trauma.

Diplopia: double vision.

Dura mater: in Latin, this literally means "tough mother"; it's the outermost covering of the brain and provides support and protection for the brain and spinal cord.

Dysarthria: speech impairment caused by inability to control the tongue or speech muscles.

Dysphagia: difficulty swallowing.

Dysphasia: inability to speak words; inability to understand spoken or written words.

Edema: swelling caused by increased fluid in and around the cells

Electroencephalogram (EEG): a recording of electrical activity in the brain by placing electrodes on the scalp. Most often used to diagnose seizures.

Embolism: a foreign body (usually a blood clot) that obstructs an artery, cutting off blood flow to the areas served by the artery.

Epidural space: the area outside the dural sac.

Epilepsy: a seizure disorder. There are many different types including grand mal (involves the whole body), focal (involves part of the body), and others.

Evoked potentials: measurement of the electrical activity of nerves.

Executive functions: the higher functions of the brain including planning, organizing, problem solving, prioritising, self-monitoring, self-correcting, and judgment.

Frontal lobe: the front part of the cerebral hemisphere containing the prefrontal (emotions, personality) and precentral (motor) areas.

Ganglia: a group of nerve cell bodies inside or outside the brain.

Glia (neuroglia): supportive cells of the brain. There are three types of glial tissue: astrocytes, oligodendrocytes, and microglia.

Glioma: any tumor arising from glial tissue.

Glial cell: one of the supporting cells of the brain.

Gray matter: areas of the brain or spinal cord consisting almost entirely of cell bodies that appear gray.

Gyrus: one of the ridges of the cerebral cortex, some of which are named.

Hematoma: a blood clot forming outside a blood vessel but within the tissues after bleeding.

Hemianopia: blindness in the same side of both eyes. This can cause an inability to see things on the left or right side.

Hemiplegia: loss of power on one side of the body.

Hemorrhage: bleeding.

Hemorrhagic transformation: bleeding that occurs in an area that was originally an ischemic stroke. The hemorrhage usually causes a worsening of symptoms.

High-density lipoprotein (HDL): "good" cholesterol since it carries cholesterol to the liver where it is broken down and destroyed.

Hydrocephalus: literally meaning "water on the brain," and usually caused by blockage of cerebrospinal fluid flow.

Hypothalamus: the area of the midbrain that controls automatic functions such as appetite, sexual rhythms, blood pressure, etc.

Increased intracranial pressure: high pressure within the skull, which can lead to brain damage if not treated.

Infarction: death of cells caused by lack of oxygen and nutrients.

Interstitial radiation therapy: implantating radioactive seeds directly into a tumor.

Ischemia: lack of sufficient blood flow to supply oxygen and nutrients to an area. If ischemia is severe enough, infarction (cell death) will occur.

Limbic system: a group of structures connected to the hypothalamus that are involved in memory, emotions, and instinctive drives.

Lobe: an area of the cerebral hemisphere. See *Frontal*, *Parietal*, *Occipital*, and *Temporal Lobes*.

Longitudinal fissure: the midline cleft separating the paired cerebral hemispheres.

Low-density lipoprotein (LDL): "bad" cholesterol; elevated levels are associated with atherosclerosis.

Lumbar puncture: a spinal tap; inserting a needle between the bones of the back to withdraw a sample of spinal fluid.

Medulla: the base of the brain stem just above the spinal cord.

Meninges: three layers of tissue covering brain and spinal cord: dura mater, arachnoid layer, and pia mater.

Meningioma: a type of brain tumor arising from the meninges.

Metastasize: to spread to another part of the body.

Neoplasm: means literally "new growth"; usually refers to a tumor.

Neuron: a nerve cell.

Nystagmus: rapid movement of the eyeballs.

Occipital lobe: the rearmost part of the cerebral hemisphere; contains areas dealing with vision.

Ommaya reservoir: a device implanted under the scalp connected to a catheter placed into a ventricle. It is used to import medications directly into the cerebrospinal fluid.

Palsy: paralysis of a single nerve or area of the body.

Paresis: muscle weakness without complete paralysis.

Paresthesia: abnormal sensations, similar to what one experiences when a foot "falls asleep."

Parietal lobe: area of the cerebral hemisphere behind the frontal lobe. Contains sensory areas and processing areas.

Pia mater: literally means "delicate mother"; this is the membrane that lies on surface of the brain and spinal cord.

Plaque: a thick deposit of fat and cholesterol in the wall of an artery caused by atherosclerosis.

Pons: part of the brain stem just above the medulla that connects to the cerebellum and contains several cranial nerves.

Postcentral gyrus: at the front of the parietal lobe; it is the primary sensory area of the brain.

Postconcussion syndrome: a group of symptoms following a head injury that can include difficulty thinking, memory loss, headache, and others. The symptoms may last for days or months.

Posttraumatic Amnesia: a period following unconsciousness when the affected person has no memory or a confused memory of events.

Precentral gyrus: at the back of the frontal lobe; it is the primary motor area of the brain.

Progressive stroke: a stroke in which symptoms worsen over time. A progressive stroke may occur because of hemorrhagic transformation, because swelling interferes with blood supply to other areas, or because further emboli have obstructed other blood vessels.

Retrograde amnesia: loss of memory of events concerning a period prior to a head injury.

Seizure convulsions: epilepsy due to temporary disruption in electrical activity of the brain.

Shoulder-hand syndrome: severe pain in the arm occurring in some people after they have had a stroke resulting in paralysis of the arm. Several problems may contribute to this condition, making treatment difficult.

Shunt: a tube that allows cerebrospinal fluid to flow from a ventricle into a body cavity. Used to relieve hydrocephalus.

Spasticity: rigidity and chronic contraction of the muscles, often caused by a neurologic disease.

Stereotactic: to be able to localize a specific point accurately in three dimensions. Stereotactic surgery uses a frame fixed to the patient's head so that a specific point deep within the brain can be found with unerring accuracy.

Subarachnoid hemorrhage: bleeding into the space within the skull but outside the brain. Common causes include aneurysm and trauma.

Syndrome of inappropriate antidiuretic hormone (SIADH): a condition where the brain abnormally secretes hormones telling the kidneys to conserve water. This can worsen cerebral edema and cause changes in the body's salt content.

Temporal lobe: the lobe of the cerebral hemisphere on the lateral side, primarily concerned with hearing and emotions.

Thrombolytic drugs: medications that dissolve blood clots.

Thrombosis: abnormal clotting of the blood within the blood vessels. Thrombosis is often involved as a cause of stroke.

Transient ischemic attack: temporary weakness, numbness, difficulty speaking, even unconsciousness that occurs when part of the brain does not receive enough blood flow. It is considered a warning sign of impending stroke.

Tremor: regular repetitive shaking movements. They may be worse at rest (resting tremor) or during an intended movement (intention tremor).

Ventricle: spaces within the brain that contain cerebrospinal fluid.

Vertebral artery: paired arteries that ascend along the spinal cord. They join together to form the basilar artery in the brainstem.

Wernicke's area: an area of the brain concerned with producing speech.

White matter: areas of the brain or spinal cord consisting almost entirely of axons and dendrites, which appear white.

Healthy Diets for Persons with Vascular Disease

Cholesterol: Maximum of 300 mg/day, but ideally less than 200 mg/day.

Total fat: Less than 30% of all calories, or less than 40 g/day.

Saturated fat: Less than 10% of all calories, or less than 12 g/day.

Cholesterol and Fat Content of Foods (per routine serving)

Food	Total Fat (g)	Saturated Fat (g)	Cholesterol(mg)
Beverages			
Alcoholic beverages	0	0	0
Coffee, black, unsweetened	0	0	0
Cafe Francais	3.4	2.9	0
Cafe Vienna	2.4	2.1	0
Irish Mocha Mint	2.6	2.2	0
Suisse Mocha	2.8	2.4	0
Juices	<0.3	0	0
Soda, carbonated drinks	0	0	0
Tea	0	0	0

Cholesterol and Fat Content of Foods (per routine serving) *continued*

Food	Total Fat (g)	Saturated Fat (g)	Cholesterol (mg)
Breads and Noodles			
Bagel	1.4	0.2	0
Biscuit	3.3	1.2	0
Bread, white or wheat	1.0	0.2	0
Cornbread	4.0	1.5	34
Crescent roll	5.0	2.7	6
English muffin	1.1	0.2	0
Kaiser roll	8.1	1.3	4
Macaroni noodles	0.4	0	0
Muffin, bran	5.1	1.8	26
Muffin, blueberry	4.3	1.3	25
Noodles, egg	2.4	0.8	50
Noodles, Ramen	6.8	1.5	0
Pancake	3.2	1.2	27
Spaghetti noodles	0.7	0.1	0
Stuffing from mix	12.2	3.0	1
Waffle, frozen	3.2	1.0	24
Candy			
Almond Joy	7.8	3.6	1
Caramels	2.9	1.3	8
Chocolate	9.0	5.0	5
Chocolate chips	12.2	6.3	1
Chocolate almonds	12.1	4.2	3
Chocolate peanuts	9.0	2.6	1
Hard candy (except butterscotch)	0.3	0	0
Jelly beans	0	0	0
Marshmallows	0	0	0
Milky Way	9.0	4.7	6
Mr. Goodbar	15.0	7.8	7
Nestle Crunch	8.0	5.0	6
Reese's Peanut Butter Cup	10.7	6.0	5
Snickers	13.0	4.4	3
Cereal			
All-Bran	0.5	0	0
Alpha Bits	0.6	0.1	0

Food	Total Fat (g)	Saturated Fat (g)	Cholesterol (mg)
Bran Flakes	0.5	0.1	0
Cap'n Crunch	2.6	1.7	0
Cheerios	1.8	0.3	0
Corn Flakes	0.1	0	0
Cream of Wheat	0.4	0.1	0
Frosted Mini-Wheat	0.3	0	0
Granola	4.9	3.3	0
Grits	0.5	0	0
Kix	0.7	0.2	0
Oatmeal	1.7	0.3	0
Product 19	0.2	0	0
Raisin Bran	0.5	0.1	0
Rice Krispies	0.2	0	0
Shredded Wheat	0.3	0.1	0
Special K	0.1	0	0
Total	0.6	0.1	0
Wheaties	0.5	0.1	0

Chips

Food	Total Fat (g)	Saturated Fat (g)	Cholesterol (mg)
Cheese puffs	10.6	2.6	1
Cheese balls, baked	6.0	1.5	1
Corn chips (Fritos)	9.7	1.6	0
Pork rinds	9.3	3.7	24
Potato chips, plain	9.8	2.6	0
Potato chips, sour cream	9.5	2.6	1
Pringles, low fat	7.0	2.0	0
Pretzels	1.0	0.5	0
Tortilla chips	7.0	1.1	0

Dairy Products

Food	Total Fat (g)	Saturated Fat (g)	Cholesterol (mg)
Butter	4.0	2.5	11
Cheese, American	8.9	5.6	27
Cheese, American, low fat	2.0	1.3	10
Cheese, cottage	5.1	3.2	17
Cheese, cottage, low fat	1.2	0.7	5
Cheese, cream	9.9	6.2	31
Cheese, mozzarella	7.0	4.4	25
Cheese, Swiss	7.8	5.0	26
Cream	2.9	1.8	10
Cream, artificial creamer	0.7	0.7	0

Cholesterol and Fat Content of Foods (per routine serving) *continued*

Food	Total Fat (g)	Saturated Fat (g)	Cholesterol (mg)
Dairy Products continued			
Cream, whipped	5.6	3.5	21
Cream, artificial			
whipped topping	0.7	0.4	2
Ice cream	23.7	14.7	88
Ice cream, low fat	14.0	8.9	59
Ice milk	5.6	3.5	18
Milk, whole	8.2	5.1	33
Milk, 2%	4.7	2.9	18
Milk, skim	0.4	0.3	4
Yogurt	7.4	4.8	29
Yogurt, low fat	3.5	2.3	14
Desserts			
Angelfood cake	0	0	0
Apple pie	11.9	4.2	4
Brownie	5.0	2.3	27
Cheesecake	14.3	8.9	30
Chocolate cake with icing	10.8	5.5	26
Chocolate chip cookie	2.3	0.9	4
Custard	7.3	3.5	154
Danish pastry	4.9	1.8	9
Doughnut	5.8	2.7	23
Doughnut, glazed	9.2	4.5	15
Eclair	15.4	7.3	195
Fig bar	1.0	0.4	6
Gelatin	0	0	0
Oatmeal cookie	3.2	1.1	13
Pecan pie	23	5.6	30
Pound cake	8.8	304	51
Sugar cookie	3.4	1.4	6
Eggs			
Egg (1)	5.6	1.7	210
EggBeater's	0	0	0
Fruit			
Apple	0.5	0.1	0
Banana	0.6	0.2	0

Food	Total Fat (g)	Saturated Fat (g)	Cholesterol (mg)
Cantaloupe	0.4	0	0
Coconut, fresh	15.1	13.4	0
Figs	0.2	0	0
Citrus fruit	0.1	0	0
Most other fruit	< 0.5	0	0

Margarine and Cooking Oils

Lard	12.8	5.0	12
Margarine	3.8	0.7	0
Oil			
Canola (rapeseed)	13.6	0.9	0
Coconut	13.6	8.1	0
Cottonseed	13.6	3.5	0
Olive	13.6	1.8	0
Palm	13.6	8.8	0
Peanut	13.6	2.3	0
Safflower	13.6	1.2	0
Sesame	13.6	1.9	0
Sunflower	13.6	1.4	0
Shortening	12.8	3.2	0

Meats (assumes lean cuts)

Beef	15-17	6.5	80
Beef liver	4.2	1.6	331
Veal cutlet	5.7	2.5	84
Bologna	8.0	3.0	16
Frankfurter	13.2	4.8	45
Fish and shellfish			
Catfish	3.6	0.8	49
Cod	0.7	0.1	47
Crab, lobster	1.5	0.2	85
Fishsticks, breaded	12.2	3.1	112
Halibut	2.5	0.4	35
Herring	9.9	2.2	65
Orange roughy	7.0	0.1	20
Oysters	2.1	0.5	47
Salmon	5.3	1.4	41
Shrimp, boiled	0.9	0.2	166
Tuna, light, in oil	7.0	1.3	15
Tuna, light, in water	0.4	0.1	15

Cholesterol and Fat Content of Foods (per routine serving) *continued*

Food	Total Fat (g)	Saturated Fat (g)	Cholesterol (mg)
Meats (assumes lean cuts) continued			
Lamb	6.9	2.3	71
Pork			
Bacon	9.4	3.3	16
Bacon, Canadian	3.9	1.3	27
Ham	9.4	3.2	80
Loin	11.8	4.1	77
Sausage	8.4	2.9	22
Poultry (Note: At least double these values if skin is left on.)			
Chicken breast	3.1	0.9	73
Chicken drumstick	2.5	0.7	71
Chicken liver	3.8	1.3	442
Chicken thigh	5.4	1.5	49
Turkey breast	0.8	0.3	73
Turkey drumstick	8.5	2.8	170
Snacks			
Cracker, saltine	0.6	0.2	2
Cracker, Ritz	2.9	0.8	5
Cracker, cheese	4.9	1.2	4
Cracker Jacks	1.0	0.1	0
Graham cracker	1.5	0.6	3
Granola bar	5.0	4.3	0
Olive, black	4.0	0.5	0
Olive, green	1.6	0.2	0
Pickle	0.2	0	0
Popcorn	0.7	0.3	0
Nuts			
Almonds	9.5	0.9	0
Cashews	13.2	2.6	0
Peanuts	14.0	1.9	0
Pecans	19.2	1.5	0
Pistachio	15.0	1.9	0
Sunflower seeds	14.1	1.5	0
Wheat Thins	1.4	0.4	2
Vegetables			
Artichoke	0.2	0	0
Avocado	27	4.5	0

Food	Total Fat (g)	Saturated Fat (g)	Cholesterol (mg)
Barley	0.5	0	0
Beans			
BBQ with sauce	4.0	1.5	1
Black-eyed peas	0.4	0.2	0
Butter	0.6	0.1	0
Garbanzo	2.4	0.5	0
Kidney	0.4	0.1	0
Lima	0.7	0.2	0
Split peas	0.3	0.1	0
White	0.6	0.2	0
Beets	0.1	0	0
Carrot	0.2	0	0
Cauliflower	0.2	0	0
Celery	0.1	0	0
Corn	0.8	0.1	0
Green beans	0.2	0	0
Mushrooms	0.2	0	0
Onion	0.1	0	0
Peas	0.5	0.1	0
Potato	0.1	0	0
Rice	0.2	0	0
Sauerkraut	0.2	0	0
Squash	0.2	0	0
Sweet potato	0.5	0.1	0
Tomato	0.3	0	0

Prepared Foods	Total Fat (g)	Cholesterol (mg)
Canned and Bottled Foods		
Chili and beans	26.0	52
Clam chowder	6.6	22
Corned beef hash	12.5	35
Salad dressings (per tablespoon)		
Blue cheese	8.0	3
French low-calorie	0.9	1
Mayonnaise, regular	11.0	8
Thousand Island	7.8	2
Soup (per cup)		
Beef broth	0.5	0
Chicken broth	1.4	1

Prepared Foods	Total Fat (g)	Cholesterol (mg)
Canned and Bottled Foods continued		
Chicken noodle	1.2	7
Cream of chicken	14.7	20
Cream of mushroom	19.0	2
Vegetable	1.9	0
Frozen Foods		
Beef enchiladas (el Charrito)	11.0	25
Beef pie (Banquet)	20.0	65
Chicken a la King (Banquet)	4.7	36
Chicken fettuccine (Healthy Choice)	4.5	40
Chicken pie (Swanson)	44.0	80
Lasagna (Stouffer)	14.0	90
Pizza, cheese (Tombstone)	19.0	50
Swedish meatballs (Budget Gourmet)	34.0	160
Restaurant Food		
Arby's		
Roast beef sandwich	15.0	39
Chicken breast sandwich	27.0	57
Fries (small)	8.0	6
Burger King		
Whopper	36.0	90
Hamburger	12.0	37
Chicken Tenders	10.0	47
Fries (small)	13.0	14
Church's		
Chicken thigh, fried	21.6	n/a
Catfish, fried	12.0	n/a
Kentucky Fried Chicken		
Chicken breast, original	17.3	96
Chicken breast, extra crispy	23.7	66
Biscuit	13.6	0
McDonald's		
Big Mac	35.0	83
Egg McMuffin	16.0	5.9
Chicken McNuggets	20.0	62
Taco Bell		
Beef burrito	21.0	n/a
Taco	34.0	n/a

Stroke Recovery
Support Groups

The best way to get up-to-the-minute information regarding strokes and to find out what techniques and support are available is through the Internet. These days, if you don't have Internet access yourself, someone you know probably does. If not, most local libraries have Internet terminals and are happy to show you how to use them. You will find many other sites by searching under "stroke," but remember—anyone can post their own Internet Web page and many for-profit companies with shady reputations do just that. I recommend that, in general, you stick to sites with "edu" (educational institutions) or "org" (nonprofit corporation) in their Web address. Sites with "com" or "net" may have very good material but are generally established by for-profit businesses.

Aneurysm & AVM Support Page
http://www.westga.edu/~wmaples/aneurysm.html
State University of West Georgia
Carrollton, Georgia 30118

Links to sites about treatment and research concerning aneurysms.

Brain Aneurysm / Subarachnoid Hemorrhage Index
http://www.uic.edu/depts/mcns/patients/angio.html
Department of Neurosurgery
Bowman Gray School of Medicine
Wake Forest University

Provides general information and a lot of links to pages concerning up-to-date treatment and diagnosis of aneurysms. Most of the linked pages are posted by individual physicians and neurology groups. Some are of general interest while others are geared more toward other physicians.

3-D Visualization of Brain Aneurysms
http://everest.radiology.uiowa.edu/DPI/nlm/apps/aneur/aneur.html

This Internet-only site has lots of pictures showing how the various tests (arteriography, MRI scan, etc.) detect aneurysms, as well as pictures of real aneurysms.

International Stroke Support & Information Web Site
http://members.aol.com/scmmlm/main.htm

On-line support complete with chat rooms for stroke survivors and their families. This is a good site to communicate with other family members who have already been through what you are going through now. While it doesn't take the place of a local support group, it could prove invaluable for people living in areas where such groups aren't available.

National Institute of Neurological Disorders and Strokes
http://www.ninds.nih.gov/healinfo/disorder/stroke/strokehp.htm
P.O. Box 5801
Bethesda, Maryland 20824
1-800-352-9424

Government agency dedicated to research also provides some written material regarding stroke. Their Web site also has dozens of articles about strokes written in understandable language.

National Stroke Association
www.stroke.org
96 Inverness Drive East, Suite I
Englewood, Colorado 80112
1-800-STROKES
(303) 649-1328 (Voice)
(800) 649-1328 (Fax)

NSA develops and distributes educational materials, a newsletter, and a stroke journal. They also operate a national clearinghouse for information, referral sources, and research as well as providing guidance for developing stroke clubs and stroke support groups. Their Web site has links to places providing assist devices, special computers, and a host of other things that make life easier after a stroke. They will send written packets to people without Internet access. Highly recommended.

Neurological Rehabilitation/Disability Index
http://www.bgsm.edu/bgsm/surg-sci/ns/stroke.html
Department of Neurosurgery
Wake Forest University School of Medicine
Winston-Salem, North Carolina 27157

This superb page has literally hundreds of links concerning stroke and aneurysm prevention, rehabilitation, and research, as well as interesting fact sheets for stroke patients. Recommended.

Stanford Stroke Center
http://www-med.stanford.edu/school/stroke/
(415) 723-4448

A superb on-line guide discussing stroke rehabilitation and treatment. For people living in the Northern California area, Stanford Stroke Center also provides medical care and rehabilitation services.

Stroke Connection/ American Heart Association National Center
7272 Greenville Avenue
Dallas, Texas 75231-4596
1-800-553-6321

The Courage Stroke Network provides a forum for sharing knowledge and experiences related to living with stroke. They also publish a useful monthly newsletter. The site is particularly useful for people who have suffered strokes and also have heart disease.

Stroke Support Group, Inc.
http://www.span.com.au/nrc/stroke_intro.html
Stroke SA Inc.
Neurological Resource Centre
23a King William Road
Unley SA 5061
South Australia

International site that is of more benefit to persons living in Canada because it is geared toward the British Commonwealth health care systems.

Brain Tumor Support and Research Groups*

Brain tumors are an area of continuing research, much of which is reported first to patients through Internet sites. These days, if you don't have Internet access yourself, someone you know probably does. If not, most local libraries have Internet terminals and will be happy to show you how to use them. You will find many other sites by searching under "brain tumor," but remember—anyone can post an Internet Web page. Specifically concerning brain tumors, a lot of pages are "infomercials" for certain techniques or medical practices. That doesn't mean they aren't reputable; the vast majority are. However, their opinion will usually be more in favor of the techniques they practice and less in favor of those they don't. For example, a site that uses a gamma knife is going to recommend that particular treatment more than chemotherapy, and vice versa.

*In addition to the sites listed here, America Online has four different discussion and on-line support groups for patients with brain tumors.

Acoustic Neuroma Association of Canada
Box 369
Edmonton, Alberta T5J 2J6
Canada

Acoustic Neuroma Association (U.S.)
Box 398
Carlisle, Pennsylvania 17013-0398

Both groups provide information and support to people with these specific types of brain tumors.

American Brain Tumor Association
http://neurosurgery.mgh.harvard.edu/abta/
2720 River Road, Suite 146
Des Plaines, Illinois 60018-4110
(847) 827-9910

They provide a newsletter, physician listings, support group listings by state, and a lot of educational material, most of which can be accessed from the Internet.

American Cancer Society
http://www.cancer.org
1-800-118-2345

Operates an informational Web page with separate sections on adult and pediatric brain tumors, provides written booklets, and offers advice and help through the 800-number listed above.

The Brain Surgery Information Page
http://www.brain-surgery.com/

Arranged to provide information to patients at New York University Hospital, the page provides invaluable information to people who are about to have surgery. A great primer on what to expect from preoperative shot to postoperative recovery.

The Brain Tumor Society
http://www.tbts.org/
1-800-770-8287
84 Seattle Street
Boston, Massachusetts 02134-1245

Extremely professional national organization that provides educational material and family support and raises funds for brain tumor research. It also helps locate support groups for individuals and families.

Brain Tumor Information Page
http://member.aol.com/lsdpout/brtmr.htm

Very helpful page accessible through the Internet, although some of its features are only available through an America Online account.

British Brain Tumour Association
http://glaxocentre.merseyside.org/bbta.html
2 Oakfield Road
Hightown, Merseyside L38 9GQ
England
0151 929 3229

Educational, information, and support for patients in the U.K.

The Compassionate Friends
http://www.compassionatefriends.org/
(630) 990-0010

This wonderful organization exists only to help grieving parents cope with the loss of a child. It has chapters in every state and throughout Canada.

Musella Foundation for Brain Tumor Research & Information
http://www.virtualtrials.com/
1100 Peninsula Boulevard
Hewlett, New York 11557
(516) 295-4740

Very informative page dedicated mostly to new advances, research, and clinical trials of brain tumor treatment. Also provides a discussion forum and links to local support groups. Includes a fair amount of "advertising" for treatment protocols. My feeling is the site is extremely useful, but you shouldn't believe everything you read without asking further questions.

National Brain Tumor Foundation
http://www.braintumor.org/faq.html
1-800-934-CURE

Provides educational seminars and support groups, although the organization is largely a fund-raising and distribution group for brain tumor research.

National Cancer Institute
http://cis.nci.nih.gov/

Provides updates on new research and operates a cancer information service.

Alzheimer's Disease Support and Research Groups

Probably more than any other topic in this book, except perhaps Parkinson's disease, the Internet is filled with resources concerning this disease. There are a host of great sites, the best of which I've tried to list here. There are also thousands of other sites, many of which are excellent.

Unfortunately, a lot of unscrupulous people are aware that Alzheimer's victims and their families are often desperate. I found a lot of sites offering ridiculous claims for herbal and ancient Eastern remedies—even voodoo cures—for Alzheimer's disease. Not all these sites are obvious sales pitches. However, many of the "informational pages" are simply fronts for people selling worthless products. Please, please be careful—any reputable site will offer free or nearly free services. If there really was an ancient Chinese herb that cured Alzheimer's disease, then why does China have just as high a rate of Alzheimer's disease as the rest of the world?

Alzheimers.com
http://www.alzheimers.com/

Very up-to-date page that contains some advertising, but also a lot of very recent information regarding newly released treatments and research studies.

Alzheimer's Disease Education and Referral (ADEAR) Center
http://www.alzheimers.org/

This government agency is a division of the National Institute on Aging, itself a department of the National Institutes of Health. The site is pretty easy to use, considering it's a government agency site and offers especially good information on new treatments and research.

The Alzheimer's Research Forum
http://www.alzforum.org/

Excellent site with links to caregiving organizations, support groups, and also a section aimed at physicians that presents a lot of information about current research. The physicians' section is probably the best site to learn about the status of investigational drugs of any Web page.

The Alzheimer's Disease Web Page
http://med-amsa.bu.edu/Alzheimer/home.html

Boston University, who administers this page, presents useful information for those caring for an Alzheimer's patient at home.

The Alzheimer's Society of Canada
http://www.alzheimer.ca/
Alzheimer Society of Canada
20 Eglinton Avenue West, Suite 1200
Toronto, Ontario M4R 1K8
Canada
(416) 488-8772
1-800-616-8816 (valid only in Canada)

Alzheimer's Disease Review
http://www.coa.uky.edu/ADReview/

Site for a journal published by the University of Kentucky. Not a complete site, but it does offer some new medical research. A word of caution, though: the articles are written in "doctorese," thus they can be a bit difficult to decipher.

The Alzheimer's Association
http://www.alz.org/
919 North Michigan Avenue, Suite 1000
Chicago, Illinois 60611-1676
1-800-272-3900
(312) 335-8700
(Fax) (312) 335-1110

The site for Alzheimer's information. The association can put you in touch with local support groups, offers a comprehensive information page, and presents links to the newest research.

The Cognitive Neurology and Alzheimer's Disease Center
http://www.brain.nwu.edu/
320 East Superior Street, Searle 11-450
Chicago, Illinois 60611-3008
(312) 908-9339
(Fax) (312)-908-8789

Northwestern University's Alzheimer's disease site. Contains some interesting information, although you have to wade through a lot of self-promotion to get to it.

Mayo Clinic Alzheimer's Resource Center
http://www.mayohealth.org/mayo/common/htm/alzheimers.htm

Very informative site with articles that strike a nice balance between being readable while still providing up-to-date information.

Parkinson's Disease Support and Research Groups

There are literally thousands of sites to be found if you search under "Parkinson's" or "Parkinsonism," far more than I found for other topics. There are also far more individual home pages devoted to Parkinsonism and a bit fewer educational sites. Individual home pages can be a great place to meet someone else who suffers from the disease. Frequently, however, they are very nonscientific sites that strongly recommend some type of treatment that really has no legitimacy.

The Mulligan Foundation
http://www.frostbyte.com/mulligan/index.html
10663 Nine Mile Road
Whitmore Lake, Michigan 48189
(313) 449-8442
(Fax) (313) 449-4931

A private foundation for Parkinsonism research. Not a lot of basic information but does have links to ongoing supported research studies.

National Institute of Health Parkinsonism Research Page
http://www.nhgri.nih.gov/DIR/LGDR/PARK2/

Not as complete as some pages but does connect to articles on recently released drug information and medication alerts.

The National Institute of Neurologic Disease and Stroke Parkinson's Information Site
http://www.ninds.nih.gov/healinfo/disorder/parkinso/pdhtr.htm

Great page for background information on Parkinsonism. Although the information is basic, and probably not as complete as that in this book, it's easy to read and well organized. This is a good site to recommend to relatives who want to learn more about the disease.

National Parkinson Foundation, Inc.
http://www.parkinson.org/
1501 NW 9th Avenue
Bob Hope Road
Miami, Florida 33136
(305) 547-6666
1-800-327-4545

Superbly organized site is full of information and very easy to maneuver in. Contains links to on-line and local support groups, to research and study information, and to centers of excellence that treat Parkinsonism.

The Parkinson Foundation of Canada National Office
710-390 Bay Street
Toronto, Ontario M5H 2Y2
Canada
(416) 366-0099
1-800-565-3000
(Fax) (416) 366-9190

Provides links to some articles and information, as well as Canadian support groups. Not nearly as much information as its American sister site, however.

Parkinson's Disease Society of the United Kingdom
http://www.sharward.co.uk/pdscont.html
215 Vauxhall Bridge Road
London, SW1V1EJ
England
0171 233 9908

Great Britain's Parkinsonism organization. The Web site contains (as of press time) very little information.

Parkinson's Disease Information Center
http://pdic.jeffreyskaye.com/

A private page, it includes information on legal rights for Parkinsonism's patients under the Americans with Disabilities Act.

The Parkinson's Institute
1170 Morse Avenue
Sunnyvale, California 94089
1-800-786-2958
(408) 734-2800

This is the Web site for an independent, not-for-profit organization conducting patient care and research. It actually started by investigating the street drug–induced Parkinsonism of the early 1980s, but has expanded to include all forms of Parkinsonism.

The Parkinson's Web
http://neuro-chief-e.mgh.harvard.edu/parkinsonsweb/Main/PDmain.
  html

Established by the Harvard department of Neurosurgery, this site contains some good background information. It also educates about the surgical procedures for Parkinsonism in detail.

PharmInfo Net
http://pharminfo.com/pin_hp.html

This Web-only site offers information about every medication available, including a complete side effect profile, drug interactions, etc.

People with Parkinson's
http://www.newcountry.nu/pd/mag.htm

This Internet-only group maintained by persons with Parkinsonism has a chat room, several Web sites, a monthly newsletter, and lots of personal support. The actual Web site address may change, but new locations can be found by searching for "People with Parkinson's."

Multiple Sclerosis Support and Information Groups

Multiple sclerosis has perhaps the best organized and most in-depth Internet support of any neurological disease covered in this book. These simply represent some of the best of literally hundreds of different support pages. There are local "real person" support groups available in almost every area, but most seem to have an Internet chat room or Web page in addition to actual meetings.

Computer Literate Advocates for Multiple Sclerosis
http://www.clams.org/
P.O. Box 10024
Bainbridge Island, Washington 98110

Provides a bulletin board and chat room for MS patients and their families, as well as links to new research, a "good doctors" list, and other helpful information.

Doctor's Guide to Multiple Sclerosis Resources
http://www.pslgroup.com/MS.HTM

This site is geared toward providing up-to-date information and news releases to doctors, but can be used by anyone. There's a bit of "med-icalese" to wade through, but it's not too bad overall.

International Multiple Sclerosis Support Foundation
http://aspin.asu.edu/msnews/imssf.htm

The IMSSF is unique in that it is run and directed entirely by volunteers with MS. Provides marvelous support including young people, children, spouses, Japanese, and Spanish bulletin boards and chat rooms. Also sponsors "Ask the Doctor" forums, has a legal assistance area, and a disability equipment swap and trade area.

Ken's Multiple Sclerosis Web Page
http://www.dcr.net/~khoward/links.htm

I rarely recommend personal pages since they tend to come and go. This very professional page, however, contains the best organized and most comprehensive set of links to MS sites I've run across.

Knowledge Weaver's Multiple Sclerosis Page
http://www-medlib.med.utah.edu/kw/ms/

Actually an on-line course about MS for medical students and physicians-in-training, it is superbly well-written and easy to understand.

MedSupport FSF International
http://www.medsupport.org/
3132 Timberview Drive
Dunedin, Florida 34698

1-800-793-0766   (Their toll-free number is staffed twenty-four hours a day.)

MedSupport FSF International is dedicated to educating and assisting people with MS, their caregivers, and their families. They host news groups on-line, publish a monthly newsletter, and provide information about MS. The Web site has good information. It's a particularly good place to find real facts that will contradict "scare press" medical articles.

The Multiple Sclerosis Society of Canada
http://www.mssoc.ca

I've included this for the sake of completeness, but the site itself contains very little information other than a means to get in touch with the MS Society of Canada.

The Multiple Sclerosis Foundation
http://www.ms.org
6350 North Andrews Avenue
Fort Lauderdale, Florida 33309
(954) 776-6805
1-800-441-7055

Huge site with an almost overwhelming amount of information. You could spend days here—literally. Everything from background information, to FDA clinical trials, to alternative medicine is here. The site is graphics intensive, so if your Internet connection is slow, you may do a lot of waiting here. It is also a bit confusing to maneuver in.

National Multiple Sclerosis Society
info@nmss.org
733 Third Avenue
New York, New York 10017
1-800-FIGHT-MS (1-800-344-4867)

Probably the best MS page overall. They provide a lot of background information, new research and news bulletins, and links to support groups. Also has in-depth discussions about every drug used to treat MS. Despite containing a lot of information, it's so well organized that you can find whatever specific topic you're interested in within seconds.

The Red Boa Society
http://139.146.233.68/boa/

Wonderful support group on-line has chat rooms, bulletin boards, annual meetings, and links to lots of useful sites. They are firm

believers in the healing power of humor and having a good time despite being afflicted with MS. If you live in the Connecticut area, it's
a must.

The World of Multiple Sclerosis
http://www.ifmss.org.uk/

U.K.–based site provides a lot of information, particularly for those
newly diagnosed with MS. It also has a lot of support and links for
those living in the U.K. and Europe.

Index

Page numbers with 'f' indicate figures and 't' indicate tables.